Flying Buttresses

A Novel of Bipolar Disorder

Flying Buttresses

A Novel of Bipolar Disorder

By

Jane Thompson

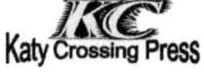

Flying Buttresses

By Jane Thompson

Published by Katy Crossing Press, LLC
Georgetown, TX
http://www.katycrossingpress.com

ISBN-13: 978-1490334257

ISBN: 1490334254

Cover art: Ross Carnes

Photographer: Ralf Kittenbacher, Artisan Photographix

Table of Contents

Marie

Carleton

Conversations

Abby

Suzy

Jackie

Missy

Marie

Carleton

Abby

Chapter One

An American exploring the Second Arrondissement of the city of Lyons, France, would smell the fragrance of flowers, see the beauty of the surrounding foothills, and find some of the oldest buildings in France. This neighborhood was built on the Presqu'île or the peninsula formed where the Saône and Rhône Rivers, which run through most of the city, come together. Included in the Presqu'île is the Cathédrale St.-Jean, a church built during medieval times, including both Romanesque and Gothic styles; its nave with its flying buttresses flinging out their support as the walls sweep toward the heavens. Besides the peninsula, the city is built on two large hills. The buildings, covered with red-tiled roofs, undulate over the hills like a drift of wildflowers.

About thirty thousand persons live in the Second Arrondissement, a town in itself. However, it contains mostly upscale shopping and the administrative offices for the city. Cafés and small shops are sprinkled throughout the neighborhood for the local residents. On the Rue Bourgelet, the American would see the National Veterinary School, the oldest veterinary school in the world. And if he were really observant, he might see a gaggle of students at a café not far from the school. The girls would all look French and speak French, so the American would probably assume they were all French students. But he would be wrong. Among them is a tall girl with a firm, straight nose, bright blue eyes, and a mass of curly, unruly black hair. While it is true she speaks fluent French, any Frenchman can tell she is American by her accent. Dressed in blue jeans and a top bought at a market down the street, the American wouldn't be able to single her out.

Abby Rachel Downs was born and raised in Connecticut. All her life, from the time she could toddle, she had a fierce love for animals. She had no fear of them and would go up to any animal to pet and hold it; she was never bitten or scratched. The pets knew she loved them. She had a special love for dogs and horses. When she was three, her parents gave her a Labrador retriever puppy, knowing it was a gentle and intelligent breed. This started a lifelong love for the dog for Abby. The rest of her life, she would have a lab at her heels. When she was older, she asked her parents for a horse.

"We can't give you a horse, Abby, they are too expensive," her mother said. She was shorter than her daughter, with straight brown hair and crinkly wrinkles around her eyes. "I know how you feel, but they have massive feed bills and you have to board them and buy tack and there are veterinarian bills and we just can't afford it. We know you really want one, but we just can't do it."

"I understand that, but I still want a horse."

"I know you do, but it is impossible. You'll just have to find a way to be around them without being able to own one. Maybe you can get a job at a stable. I never told you this, but that's what I did when I was a teenager."

By the time she was an adolescent, Abby made up her mind to be a veterinarian and to take care of horses, but meantime she had to satisfy her love for them by taking a job at a local stable, just like her mother, mucking out stalls and exercising the horses when needed; all for minimum wage. The stable rented out riding horses, and Abby helped to keep the horses clean and groomed. She also worked to keep them fed and watered. The horses knew her and responded to her with affection. It was not a glamorous job by any stretch of the imagination, but it made Abby happy.

Abby did well in high school, finishing in the top ten of her graduating class. It was a smaller school, with only about five hundred students, but she stood out, taking as much science and math as was available to her. She fulfilled her language requirements with French and she loved French history. Also, Advanced Placement tests would help to get her ahead of the game when she would get to college. She dated several guys, but nothing was serious. With her eyes set on college and then vet school, nothing was going to get in her way.

After high school graduation, she was accepted at the University of Connecticut Storrs Campus. The first thing she did after unpacking and orienting herself to the campus was to make an appointment with a counselor. Walking over to the Counseling Office, she admired the older large red and buff brick buildings interspersed with grey and white stone ones. Of course, there were newer buildings with sweeping glass façades. It looked just like a college should. When she arrived at the counselor's office, she told her, "I am determined to go to vet school. I need your help to develop a curriculum that will get me there. That's all I have ever wanted to do."

The counselor was a middle-aged black woman, Ms. Walker, who had seen just about every kind of student come through her office. She was a little startled by Abby's determination.

"Well, I don't always see students who are so certain of what they want to accomplish. You seem quite sure of yourself." Using her computer, she looked up Abby's records. "I see you have tested out of several of the basic freshman courses. That means you have a head start on some of the technical classes you need to take. Let me pull up the necessary courses for veterinary school and we'll make a plan for the next four years that'll get you where you want to go."

Abby signed up for the classes the counselor recommended and started working toward her goal. She had fun in college, dating and going to parties and dances, but, again, never lost sight of that goal. She had to work part-time to help pay for school, but also went to summer school to get in some extra classes. In summer school, she concentrated on her French language classes. She was able to finish her undergraduate classes in three years, magna cum laude.

Several months before graduation, her counselor, Ms. Walker, met with her,

"Abby, you have done everything you can to ready yourself for veterinary school. Now we start the fun part, applying to schools. Have you thought about where you want to go?"

"My first choice is Virginia Tech, and I know Texas A&M is good, too. But I really prefer Tech because it has such a good reputation and is closer to home."

"I suggest you apply to both those schools and to a couple more, including right here at the University. Let's get started and give you a chance to hear by June." Ms. Walker got all the applications for her and made sure Abby had all the papers and the references she needed and in good time. Then they sat back and waited.

Close to graduation, she came back to her room to find her roommate, Sandy, studying for finals. Sandy, who was short, blond, and plump, had become her best friend during their first year at school. They had spent many evenings in conversations about their beliefs and values and found that they had much in common. Both were feminists who wanted to be the star in their own lives. Sandy, who wanted to be a lawyer, decided that Abby had the right idea about getting through undergraduate school as fast and as painlessly as possible, followed her lead and also finished school in three years. "Abby, I am so glad I had your example to follow. It really is a waste of time and money to spend four years getting a BA. Now I can go straight to law school, having saved my parents and me a lot of money. Don't think they haven't appreciated it."

"My sister, who is brilliant, did the same thing and gave me the idea. I'm glad we got through it," answered Abby.

Now, seeing her studying so hard, Abby hated to interrupt her, but she had to ask, "Sandy, did you check the mail today?"

Sandy didn't look up. She said, "Hmmm? Yes."

Abby said, "Well, I wonder when I am going to get a letter from one of the schools? This is driving me nuts."

"Oh, Abby, I forgot! You did get a letter today. And I meant to give it to you the minute you came in the door. I can't wait to see what it says."

Sandy pulled the crinkled-up letter from her purse. It was from Virginia Tech, Admissions Office. Abby said, "Sandy, open it. I haven't got the nerve."

Sandy opened it up and shrieked. Abby grabbed it from her, saw the acceptance, and jumped up and down. "Oh, Sandy, this is great! I don't have to worry and wait anymore, and I don't have to open any more letters! I got my first choice."

Abby called her parents. "Guess what! I got into Virginia Tech, and I got a tuition scholarship! That will help a lot. I am so excited."

"Abby, that's great. We hoped you would go to Tech since you wanted it so badly, and yes, the scholarship is a big help. We are so glad for you. We'll see you at graduation next month. We can't wait to see you with that special honor stole," her mother said.

Chapter Two

Abby spent the summer between undergrad and vet school working two jobs so she could pay for as much of her schooling as possible. She knew vet school would be difficult, but she was so excited about going she wasn't worried and could hardly wait. Leaving Cassie, her lab, so far behind would be difficult and she wouldn't be able to visit the horses so often. She was looking forward to making new animal friends, and could visit the old ones on vacations.

She hit the ground running at Virginia Tech, but soon found that vet school was harder than she realized. It was like going to medical school, only with different kinds of patients. Abby made friends fast; people were just automatically drawn to her. She went to some upper class friends and asked,

"What tricks do you know for keeping up? I am floundering here; I've always done well in school. I don't know what to do."

Pam, a pretty brunette who kept her hair back in a knot, skewered, said, "Yes, it is scary at first. You don't think you will ever get the hang of it. I'll show you how I've learned to take notes and how I prioritize. Some of the other girls will help, too."

Abby followed her advice and was soon getting along better in her classes. She didn't have a lot of animals to practice on at first and that was disappointing; but she did make friends with as many animals she could on campus. She was just learning the basics. That was hard. Things began to come a little easier, and she started to catch on. Her grades improved, and Abby climbed back into the top ranks of her class. By the end of the year, she was right up there with the best, and working to stay there. Vet school bore little relationship to undergrad school, and she had to learn to budget her time and get as much work done in as little a time span as possible. She was never much of a procrastinator and learned to never put anything off in graduate school. As soon as she got an assignment, she had to set it up and/or outline it so her brain could start working on it. There was only a little time to socialize, but she did as much of that as she could, being the gregarious person she was.

The next summer was just like the first; two jobs to keep her in school. It was a grind, but it was living her dream. The second year of vet school was even harder than the first. She caught on to the how-to-accomplish-its of the school, but it was still just a lot of work. At the end of the school year, she was exhausted. Abby went home with no thought to her summer plans at all. Maybe she would just work with the horses and try to relax. Her parents had other plans, though. Her mom and dad sat her down the day after she got home, after letting her sleep in. Her dad, who was tall and lean, brushed his hand through his black, curly hair, sat in his brown, corduroy-covered easy chair while her mom and Abby relaxed on the brown and black patterned couch.

"Abby, you have worked so hard the past few years, and you have certainly got good results. I can tell just by looking that you are really tired out. I had a good year and got an outstanding bonus. Nothing would make me happier than if you would spend the summer in France. I know you have always wanted to go."

Abby was speechless. At first, the only thing she could think of to say was, "Really?"

Then she caught her breath and exclaimed, "Thank you. That would make me happier than anything. It would be a complete change from school."

[7]

"We will miss you, but we know that visiting France has always been your dream and I can't think of anything that would take your mind off your studies more. Make your reservations as fast as you can so you can enjoy as much of the summer as you can there."

"Oh, Dad...."

"Scoot."

Abby ran upstairs to her room, which was generally tidy but right now had suitcases and clothes dribbled around it. It had yellow-flowered wallpaper, white drapes, and white furniture. Immediately, she started to straighten it up, partially to calm herself down with rote work, and partially so she could sit down and plan her trip in a neat room. Actually, Abby didn't have to plan much. She had dreamed of a trip to France so often that she already knew where she wanted to go and what she wanted to see. She made a reservation for the plane in two days departing from New York to Paris, and then just assumed she would get around by train, winging it from there. After Paris, she wanted to see the hedgerows in Normandy. This was true ever since her grandfather, who fought in them in World War II, told her about them. She was especially interested in the South of France, and decided to go where her feet took her once she got there.

Abby bought a big soft bag and packed it with tops, jeans, one nice dress, and a hat. She checked with her parents to make sure they could take her to New York City to catch her plane, and then made sure she had an up-to-date guide to consult. She was ready. Her French was good and she was eager to explore the country. It didn't occur to her to worry about anything. She was supremely confident in her abilities.

Her parents drove her to New York to catch her plane and hugged her goodbye—hard. "We have never been apart as long as we will be this summer. We will miss you, but we know it will be good for you and how much you are looking forward to it. Take care of yourself and know we are thinking of you," said her mother.

Abby waved "bye" and didn't look back. When she arrived in Paris, metro and train schedules were her first targets. Her intention was to do Paris right away—all the places she had read about and longed to see. Then she would take off and see the rest of the country.

So of course, it was Versailles, the Louvre, and the other, less-known sights. She had already pictured them in her mind; but in reality, they exceeded her expectations. She was brought to tears by the artistry of what she saw at the Louvre and Versailles, the classic tourist sites. She had to see Notre Dame. The lacy architecture and the incomparable stained glass windows took her breath away. She found it difficult to tear herself away from the sights, but when she did, she went out and noticed how it looked on the outside. Again, the architecture was beautiful, and Abby realized the delicate building was held up by the sweeping props, strong flying buttresses, that supported the walls. They looked so inconsequential, but they were what made all that beauty possible.

Abby tore around Paris as if she could never see enough, but after three weeks a longing to see the countryside swept over her so she made the trip to Normandy. She was overcome by its beauty but also by the way it exactly matched the image her grandfather conveyed to her. The sunken roads, the hedged, enclosed fields were already in her mind. They looked just as she envisioned them, but even more picturesque. After Normandy, she just started sightseeing, going where it felt right, traveling by train and staying with people she met or at youth hostels, where she met others to travel with. She was friendly and outgoing, and started conversations by saying, "I'm an American; where are you from?"

They would answer, and Abby would follow up with questions about their country, always trying to learn as much as possible. Eventually, she would be peppered by questions about America and tales about visits there. Making friends quickly, Abby had no problems finding places to stay. Abby was careful with the money her parents gave her, hoping she could return some of it to them at the end of the summer.

With only a month of the summer left, Abby traveled to Lyons. The city immediately entranced her, seeming to her to be less impersonal and smaller than Paris. She started exploring it, and was especially interested in touring the National Veterinary School, the oldest vet school in the world. She heard about it at Tech, and here she was in the same town. So after orienting herself to the city, one of the first things Abby did was to show up at the school and ask for a tour. One of the admissions staff showed her around, and Abby was impressed. Everything was hospital-clean and the animals were receiving the best of care. The horses were lined up in a long row of stalls, with every conceivable kind of tack and equipment to care for them in the building. The woman who showed her around, a middle-aged lady with a few wrinkles but with the French allure so common among the women of the country, was impressed with Abby's knowledge and her command of French. She asked Abby if she would like to meet the academic Dean, and Abby was delighted.

She dressed tastefully for her appointment, even going out and buying a new dress for it. The Dean was an older man with grey hair and a little moustache. He sat in an office paneled in walnut, furnished with a tasteful wooden desk and lined with old books. He was interested in Abby's studies at Tech, and told her how the school was run in Lyons.

"Abby," he said, "I called Tech and checked up on you. You are an excellent student and you certainly know your French. It is not widely known, but there are full scholarships available to foreign students to study here. I would like to offer you one of these scholarships. You wouldn't have to pay anything except your rent and food. The school considers it a plus to have students of differing cultures studying here."

Abby gasped, shocked at the opportunity. She could go to vet school and immerse herself in the French culture at the same time. She loved being in France and wanted to stay as long as possible. When she got her breath back, she said, "What an honor you are offering me. I would have to talk to my Dean at Tech, and, of course, my parents, but I am thrilled at the thought. I could spend more time here while attending the oldest and one of the best veterinary schools in the world. How much time would you give me to think about it?"

"We just need enough time to get you set up for the scholarship. We would want to know just a week before school starts in the first week of September. So you think about it and let us know."

"Thank you, Dean de Combrey. I will let you know my decision as soon as possible." Abby fairly floated out of his office, not thinking at all, but feeling that she had been given an opportunity she never expected.

.

Chapter Three

Abby spoke with the Dean at Tech, and he saw nothing wrong with her studying for a year in France, so long as the required courses were taken. She got on the phone with her father, telling him: "Dad, you won't believe what happened. I was offered a full scholarship to the vet school here in Lyons. I would only have to pay room and board. You know it is the oldest vet school in the world and it has a tremendous reputation. Please let me take it."

Her father sounded surprised and a little taken aback. "Abby, it means we wouldn't see you until next summer. We would miss you so much."

"And I would miss you two. But this kind of opportunity only comes once in a lifetime. It would be great for my career and I would also get to know so much more about France and its culture. Why don't you ask Mom what she thinks?"

"Well, of course I'll talk it over with your mother. We'll expect you to call us back tomorrow night. We'll have a decision for you by then."

Abby was over eighteen; her parents couldn't really keep her from taking the scholarship.

Of course, she wanted their approval and it would help to have their financial support. She walked around in a daze all day, wondering what they would say. That night she called them back, and her mother answered. "Hi, Abby, it's so good to talk with you. We've talked it over and while it will be hard on us, we know you just can't pass it up. It's not that long until summer and while we will miss you, it is too good an opportunity not to take it. Both Dad and I are happy for you."

"Thank you both. I am happy, and I promise to write often and we can talk on the phone. I love you."

When Abby got to Lyons, she moved into a hostel. She preferred hostels to hotels, mainly because they were so much cheaper, but also because they were so much more informal. True, she had to sleep in a bunk bed in a dormitory and she had to share the bathroom, but it was a good way meet other travelers and learn about their adventures, and she had a base from which to explore the city.

When she fundamentally knew her way around, she logged on to the website for student housing and found a cozy room in a home where students could live with a family close to the school. The room was small, but would meet all of her basic needs and the family even provided some meals. The room had a sunny window and a desk in the corner for studying. The rent was affordable, and Abby could borrow a bicycle for free from the street bicycle stands if her ride was less than fifteen minutes. That gave her plenty of time to get to and from school. Two of her requirements, housing and transportation, were managed quickly and easily.

She spent the few weeks left before school started in intensive study of the French terms needed for classes. A little café was sited just a block from the school. It was homey and many of the veterinary students went there for coffee and meals between classes. She met students there and told them she would start school next term and asked for their help. They were eager to help her.

"Here is a list of books for next term. I will make a copy and bring it to you tomorrow. All the words you need to know are in those books and some of them have a lexicon," one of the boys, Guy, answered.

The other students gathered around, eagerly asking questions about her background and her schooling in the

United States. Laughingly, she said, "Slow down, I can only answer one question at a time." Then they asked their questions more slowly and she described Virginia Tech and the schooling there, and how she got to France.

When she got the copy of the list of books, she bought them all and devoured them, hoping that would give her a leg up on her studies. When school started, it was just like Tech, and Abby fitted in right away. Lyons was her town, she decided, and she loved the school.

One of the girls she met in the café and later in classes was Simone Sagan, who was tall like Abby. She was always tossing back her long, smooth brown hair and she had the blue eyes of a French woman. Optimistic and intelligent, Simone began their relationship when they met in the café by asking, "What is veterinary school like in America?"

Abby told her how the two schools differed, but explained to her that they weren't really different because she attended one of the best schools in the States, Virginia Tech. "The facilities in both schools are state-of-the art, and the teachers seem like the best."

"The major differences I can see is that here you speak French."

"I would think that you would have a problem with that."

"No, I am lucky. I picked it up fast in high school and college plus when I got here, some of the other students went out of their way to help me learn the French words that I would need in school. I am going to love it here, I can tell."

"And I love that you are here. We can study together and you can tell me about America. All I know is what I have seen in the movies," said Simone.

"Then you need an education, and I need a study partner.'

Over time, as the two women worked together and talked about their respective countries, they became best friends. Abby was invited to her parent's home where she continued her education about France and how the average person in France lived. Simone's family lived in an apartment in Paris, and when she went there the family took her to places in Paris she never would have known of just using her guide. She was overwhelmed by the beauty of the places they showed her, such as the architecture of private homes and the small, private, jewel-like gardens of their friends. She showered her thanks on them, "I can't believe I saw all those beautiful places. Thank you so much."

"You can do the same when Simone comes to America," said her mother.

"I would love it if Simone came to America, and I would show her around as best I could. You know America is a lot bigger than France."

"Next time you must come to our summer place in Provence."

"Oh, that will be wonderful, I can hardly wait. Right after school is out, before I go home." But Abby never got to make that trip.

Abby started classes and was soon gratified to learn that she was able to keep up. Simone helped her a lot, but her French was good and the course work wasn't harder than at Tech. Her professors were excellent, and ranged from the young to the almost elderly. One of her professors, the one who specialized in horses, took an interest in Abby because she was also absorbed with horses. He basically took her under his wing. They talked after class about the subject matter and especially about horses. She had question after question and he answered them all, not minding teaching her all she wanted to know. After a while, they starting meeting for drinks in a small bistro away from the campus in the evenings to continue their conversations, and they didn't always talk about horses there.

After all of Abby's diligent focus all those years, she found herself falling in love with the dark, light-eyed Philippe Riboud, a Frenchman who looked the part. She was surprised at herself; she had never done anything like this before. Philippe began to represent all the men she had longed to be with all the years she concentrated on her studies. He said, "Abby, you are beautiful. I can't believe that you have come into my life. It is so rare to meet an American with your depth and understanding. You are more French than American. I understand you perfectly."

She started to not care he was married. When he suggested they meet some night in the suburbs at a hotel, she didn't turn him down. The sex was explosive and she could not resist him anymore. They met every night he could get away to the suburbs, taking the train separately. Within a few weeks, Abby was obsessed with him. Sex with him was different than it had ever been before—she had never known sex that lifted her so high or that she craved so intensely. She couldn't wait to meet him again between trysts. Her grades dropped some, but still, she was enough of a good student to keep her grades high enough to continue to qualify for her scholarship.

Philippe was besotted with her and promised her repeatedly that he would leave his wife and children for her at the end of the school year and go to America with her. They found it difficult to keep their hands off each other during the school day. They were sure they were keeping their liaison a secret from everyone, even though anyone looking at them could see their love for each other in their eyes.

When Christmas break came, Abby sent cards and lovingly selected presents to her family and friends, things they would treasure because they were French and from her, but she really didn't miss home as much as she anticipated. She had Philippe, though of course they couldn't see each other on Christmas Day because he had to spend it with his family. He said, "Abby, my love, we will never spend another Christmas apart, I swear to you." Abby was never happier.

After the holidays, Abby went back to school and her grades began to improve as she looked forward to the end of the term. It is true that she would return to America in the spring, but Philippe would return with her. After his divorce was final, they would marry and they could work together for the rest of their lives. Abby had never had a relationship like this one and she knew he was the love of her life, her soul mate. She planned to surprise her parents with Philippe, so she didn't tell them about him in her letters and phone calls home. Until he left his family, it was not a done deal even though she had complete faith in him.

As spring arrived, she noted that he did not seem to want to make any concrete plans for their future. He kept putting her off. Finally, when it became obvious that she was being stonewalled, the ultimatum was given: either make plans or break up with her. Philippe answered, "I cannot do it, Abby, I cannot leave my wife until my children are out of school. They are only six and eight. They are too young for me to leave them. I hope you understand and you will wait for me that long. You can stay and work in France and we can continue our relationship."

Abby was devastated. She broke into tears and beat on his chest with her fists. "Philippe, how could you do this? I believed you. I love you."

She had been so happy and it turned out he was stringing her along. She confided in her friend, Simone, who came to her room when Abby didn't show up at class the next day. They sat on the bed with the ivory-colored bedspread and Simone told her she wanted to disclose this to her months before, but didn't think Abby was ready to hear it. "Abby, he has done this before. He chooses someone who doesn't know his history, and turns on the charm. I wish I had felt free to warn you about him. I thought it would end this way."

Abby was angry with Simone for not telling her the facts, but in her heart she knew Simone was right—she wouldn't have listened to her. He hadn't loved her, after all his pretty words. Abby was just the typical French mistress. She was angry and sad at the same time. She also felt extremely stupid for falling for the oldest line in the world. At first she just stayed in her room and cried, but the second day, Simone came back and asked her, "Abby, are you going to let this useless man end your lifelong dream?"

Abby hung in by sheer force of will and got through her finals. Then, without a backward glance, returned to her parent's home in Connecticut. They met her at the airport, hugging her hard and happy that she was home. They did not know how to react to her mood. "Abby, what's wrong with you?" Her mother pled, asking her to confide in her while they unpacked in Abby's yellow and white bedroom.

"Mother, I had a bad relationship in France. I thought I would be over it now, but I can't seem to stop thinking about it. I'm sure I'll get over it soon. Just give me a little space and time."

She expected to be unhappy, but not so anxious or unable to rest or as obsessed as she turned out to be. She couldn't rest or relax and couldn't stop thinking about Philippe. Her parents were no help; they just didn't understand. They had no idea the relationship with him was so intense, and didn't know how to help her get through it. Crying and pacing, Abby stayed up all night and couldn't finish anything she started.

Finally, she called Sandy, her old roommate from college, and poured out her heart. Sandy was upset to hear that Abby was so unhappy and unsettled, but immediately made a decision. Sandy had finished law school at Southern Methodist University and now had a good job with Trammel Crowe. She had a two-bedroom apartment in University Park, one of the most desirable parts of Dallas. She told Abby, "just pack up your stuff and come stay with me. We'll have a good time together."

Abby decided that sounded better than staying home all summer, so she did just that. She flew to Dallas and moved in with Sandy, who completely understood. The apartment was nice, and Abby had her own bedroom and bath. That way Abby and Sandy could keep their distance.

However, Abby brought her problems with her and things did not improve. "Sandy, I have to tell you what happened. In France, while I was going to school, I fell in love with one of my professors. He paid a lot of attention to me and made me feel really special. He made promises to come to America with me and we would start a practice together. At the end of the school year, I found out that he was lying and had no intention of leaving his wife. I know the relationship is over with, but I keep obsessing over him and wanting to return to France to be with him."

"I'm so sorry that happened, but you aren't the first woman that happened too. You need to suck it up and get over that turkey. He sounds like a real jewel."

"I know, I'll try."

After a few weeks, Sandy, who had some experience with mental illness in her family with a cousin who had bipolar disorder, thought she knew what Abby should do. Sandy was close to her cousin when they were teenagers, and could recognize the signs. She talked Abby into making an appointment with the Mental Health Center for some counseling.

Abby met her doctor, Dr. Montgomery, at the rundown, depressing Mental Health Center. He listened to her story and evaluated her symptoms. The doctor said, "You are depressed, but that is part of a bigger picture. You have bipolar disorder; that is part of what allowed you to have that laser-like focus in your life when you were reaching for a goal. It is also what caused you to fall in love so completely, and now makes you obsess about that departed loved one. We need to get you on some medication to elevate your mood, but also to stabilize your moods. It may take a while to get you on the right meds, but all these anxiety and obsessive symptoms will go away. I promise."

"I hope it happens soon, as I need to get back to school in the fall."

"I want to get you stable by then. Let's start today with a couple of medications I think will help. Come back in two weeks and we'll see how you are."

"Okay, Doctor, I'll give it a try. I'm not sure I can go to school in this condition."

Suzy

Chapter Four

S uzy Clare Fontaine was dirty, her face, hands, and her clothes. She was smelly. She smelled old, and a little rotten. She hadn't bathed in nearly two weeks. She was going to have to arrange a visit to her parent's house when her father wouldn't be there so she could take a bath. She was sure there weren't any cameras there.

Suzy was small and slight, with light brown hair, a turned-up nose, and a freckled face. She was cute more than pretty, but the worried look she had on her face disguised that. Her fingernails were bitten to the quick. She mostly wore jeans and a t-shirt with a rocker's name on it.

At her house, she smashed the cameras she knew about with a hammer. However, that didn't take care of the ones that she didn't know the location of. They might be anywhere. And she was careful about what she said because of the microphones. People were watching and listening to her.

She didn't know why they were watching and listening, but she knew in her bones they were out there. She couldn't afford for them to get anything on her, so she was cautious. When her father asked her why the smoke alarms were smashed, she said it was an accident. He said, "I'll replace them right away."

"No, please don't. I want them that way."

"What?"

"I want them to stay the way they are. Please don't change them."

"But what if there is a fire?"

"I'll know, but I don't need those to tell me. Just leave it alone, please, father?"

"Okay, but I don't understand it."

Jane Thompson

Suzy hated having to argue with her father. He paid her house payment and her utilities, leaving her with just her truck payment, food, and clothes to manage. She knew he wouldn't believe her if she told him there were cameras and microphones in the house, so she just didn't mention it to him. Her mother didn't understand, either, but she was willing to go along with what she called "Suzy's quirks." She was diagnosed with bipolar disorder, but her medications didn't seem to be helping much. Suzy didn't care; she lived in her own world.

She stayed up all night and slept all day. The only time she left the house was to go to the grocery store or shopping for clothes, or to get gas. She worried constantly about money. How would she ever make it? Suzy was on disability, and didn't do much for herself. She mainly felt fear and loss. She had a relationship with a fringe rock star and she was obsessed with that. He, Emmanuel Sanchez, came to play at her sister's club. Suzy met him and instant attraction happened.

"Emmanuel, I can't believe I went to bed with you so soon after meeting you," she said, lying back on the pillow.

"Call me Manny. Sometimes things just work out that way. You and I were meant to be together. Nothing will keep us apart."

He really cared about her and kept in touch with her afterward. Two weeks after they met, he bought her a plane ticket to Kansas City, where he was booked. She felt like a star herself as she watched the show from backstage. It was weird, seeing how utilitarian everything was behind the curtains, how nothing was meant to be glamorous there, just dusty wooden floors, and plain chairs, but beyond the curtain everything was meant to look beautiful. Afterwards, she went to eat with Manny and the band. They were in a good, relaxed mood and Manny introduced her, "This is

Suzy. You are going to be seeing a lot of her. So you better like her."

Shyly, Suzy said "hello." She didn't say much after that, but drank everything in. She wanted to save every memory in her mind, knowing that something like this might never happen again. She got telegrams from him from every place he played, and she was always excited to hear from him. He usually just made a crack about the theatre or the town where he was booked, but he always signed off with "Love." He sent her flowers a couple of times.

Three weeks after the KC trip, he called and invited her to an Oklahoma City show, to be followed up by a show in Tulsa. Of course, she said "yes" and happily flew to Oklahoma City on a ticket he bought for her. He met her at the airport, "Hey, it's great to see you. I've missed you."

"I have missed you too. Do you ever think we can get together when there isn't a show involved? Just the two of us?"

"Maybe so. We'll just have to see how our schedules work out."

Again, Suzy watched from the wings, taking in all the things she didn't know about the inner workings of show business. Afterwards, she again went to dinner with Manny and the band, but this time Manny said, "It's an early night for us, guys. Got to get on that plane for Tulsa in the morning so we can make an early sound check and then relax before the show."

He took Suzy to his room along with a bottle of champagne. They drank a little and slowly made love in the king-sized bed. He made her feel special and cared for, and she was in love with him. She assumed, from his treatment of her, he loved her too. The next morning they rose early, had breakfast, and caught a short flight to Tulsa. When they got to their hotel, Manny told her, "We have to go to sound check and will be gone for a couple of hours. Maybe you can go swimming or shopping."

"No, I don't want to be away from you that long. Why can't I go? I won't get in the way, I promise."

"It's a work thing and we just don't need you there. Find something to do and I'll be back in no time."

"Oh, please let me go with you."

"No, and that's all there is to it. I want you to do what I tell you."

Manny walked away and didn't look back. Suzy threw herself on the bed and started to cry. Eventually she fell asleep and when she woke up, Manny was back. "You see, I wasn't gone long and you didn't have to go through that boring thing. Now let's get something light to eat before the show."

"Manny, I'm so glad you are back. I missed you."

Again, that night she enjoyed the show, though the edge was off her pleasure. She felt uneasy about the difference of opinion she had with Manny earlier, but tried not to let it bother her. She was a guest of a rock star at a show where people came to hear him sing and to listen to his new songs. She was backstage and watching all the action. She didn't know how she could have a better deal. Tonight she would laugh and joke as she had supper with his band and him, and then she would sleep with him in his fancy room at the hotel. No, there was nothing wrong with her life.

Chapter Five

Manny sent her back to Dallas with the usual "I love you," but there were no flowers waiting for her when she arrived. She looked up his schedule on his website and saw that he was busy, and that's what she told herself when she didn't hear from him the for a week. When another week went by, she tried to call him.

She got his manager, who said, "Hi Suzy, what's happening?"

"I hadn't heard from Manny in a couple of weeks and I wondered if he was okay."

"Oh, yeah, he's fine. Caught a little cold and he's been trying to save his voice. That's probably why he hasn't called you. Don't worry about it, luv."

"Okay, thanks."

Suzy felt better after that conversation. After two more weeks, she assumed his cold was better, but she hadn't heard from him. Again, she called, and again she got Trey, the manager. "I know he's been meaning to call, but he's just been that busy. I'll tell him you called, luv." He hung up the phone.

Suzy did not feel better after that call, but knew he couldn't have just stopped loving her. It was true that there were all these pictures of him in the magazines with different girls, but that was just for publicity. He didn't care for any of them and told her so himself. It was her he loved.

Suzy waited, but was not patient about it. She kept checking his website and wouldn't leave the house for fear he might call and she would miss it. When she ran to the grocery store, she took the phone off the hook so he would get a busy signal. However, he never called

She called Trey again, but this time he just said, "Haven't got time to talk with you now, catch you later."

Suzy's frustration was mounting. She had to find a way to get through to Manny. She knew he still cared for her, but something was keeping them apart. Then she thought of his fan page on his website. She hadn't even registered on it because she didn't feel like a fan; she was his lover. Now she registered, with a user name he would recognize, and left him a message that would be meaningful to him.

The next morning she ran straight to her computer and booted up, but there was no reply. At least it hadn't been deleted. She waited two more days, then, frantic, she left a message. "Manny, please remember the nights we spent together and times you told me you loved me. You are so dear to me, please call me and we can talk just as we used to."

She left that message around three in the morning and sat in front of the computer waiting for something to happen. She drank coffee the whole morning until nine, when she refreshed the website and saw that her message had disappeared. She cried aloud and then tried to post another message; this time her user name wouldn't take. Nor would another. She wasn't allowed to post on his fan site anymore.

"Oh no," Suzy said aloud. "Manny, how could you do this to me? You know how much I love you." Suzy shut down the computer and cried the rest of the day. At least she didn't have to wait for a phone call anymore, though she could always hope that he might change his mind, miss her, and call.

She found that she could still read the entries on the fan page, but not initiate or reply to any of them. This frustrated her to no end, especially when she realized that his last song was written about her. It was such an honor to have him write a song for her, but she couldn't discuss it with him or on his fan page. She was so proud of it.

It was shortly after this that the cameras and microphones appeared in her home. She didn't know if it was Manny watching out for her or if it was someone hired by him to make sure she stayed in line. All she knew was that it scared her. She wrote letters to Manny, asking him to stop the surveillance, but did not hear from him. It was just that he must still be interested in her, if he was willing to go to those lengths to keep track of her. Maybe he just didn't want her to talk about him, so she was careful not to do so in her home. It was scary to think she was being watched. Several times she addressed the cameras, "Manny, you can call me anytime, but you don't need to watch or listen to me. I still love you and I wouldn't do anything to hurt you." No response.

She wanted to share all the details of the relationship, so when she went to the Mental Health Center she could tell the people how Manny wrote his last song for her, and how she used to travel with him and the band, and all the flowers and notes he sent her. She would say, "I haven't heard from him in the past six months, but he has so much to do. You know, he writes all his own songs and then he has to record them; that takes more time than you would think. Then he has to promote them by appearing on TV and going on tour. I know I will hear from him soon, I'm just not sure when."

The women would ask questions, "Is he as good-looking in person as he is on TV? How tall is he? Is he nice? Where did he take you? How was he in bed?"

Suzy would answer all their questions, even telling them he was "good in bed." However, after she had satisfied their curiosity and answered all their questions, they weren't interested anymore. They wanted to move on to new topic of conversation, and Suzy would not. She persisted in talking about Manny, and soon she was sitting alone. Manny was the only thing Suzy was interested in talking about and she couldn't understand why the others blew her off.

When Dr. Wilson, who was tiny and had long, curly black hair, called her in for her appointment at the Mental Health Clinic, she asked her, "Suzy, how long has it been since you have had a bath?"

Suzy answered, "Not long, maybe a couple of days."

"I think it has been longer than that."

Suzy shrugged. "Maybe."

"What have you been doing with your time?"

"Not much, mostly just waiting for Manny to call or write."

"How long has it been since you have heard from him?"

"It's been about six months, but I know he will come back to me. He really loves me. He's just been really busy lately."

"I don't think the meds you are taking now are doing the trick. You are taking your meds?"

"Well, mostly, when I remember."

"Do you have a pill container with the days of the week on it?"

"No, I don't."

"Here's one. Put your pills in here on a night when you always watch a certain TV show or do or eat something special. That will remind you to load your pillbox. Then you will have them arranged conveniently for you to take. Try it. You will find it will be much easier to remember.

Also, I'm changing your antidepressant to Zoloft now that it has a generic and raising the dosage of the others. When you come back next month, I want to see you doing better."

"All right, I'll try. I really have been pretty unhappy the past few months."

Chapter Six

Embarrassed, Suzy realized that if her doctor could recognize that she wasn't bathing from across the desk, then a lot of people knew. Her sister, Martha, who was a successful lawyer besides owning a club, said something to her about it, but Suzy thought she was just teasing. Horrified at herself, Suzy arranged with her mother to bathe at her place that afternoon. When she got home, she gathered up all the clothes that had accumulated over the past weeks and washed everything. Then she went to the drugstore and got her meds, and when she got home, she carefully portioned out the meds in her new pillbox for the next week.

For the next two weeks, Suzy concentrated on staying clean and on doing what she could to clean up the house. That was impossible, since she saved everything she ever owned and it was piled up in all the rooms. She didn't throw anything away, but she did rearrange it somewhat. The small house was dark, because Suzy kept the curtains and shades drawn all the time. The furniture had belonged to her family, so it was formal, French provincial style; something that she would not have picked for herself. Her belongings were stacked and piled on every surface; mostly it was books she couldn't let go of. She kept the kitchen mainly clear so she could cook a little and eat.

She found that as she concentrated on these other tasks, she didn't completely obsess about Manny. She thought about him a lot, but she was able to think about other things, too. Her world brightened up some, and she didn't worry so much about the cameras and microphones. As a matter of fact, she began to wonder if anyone was really monitoring them. Perhaps they only looked in on her occasionally. Though it frightened her some, after a month

Suzy was able to bathe in her own house again. She picked times when she knew Manny was onstage or busy, not wanting to miss his phone call. She was washing her clothes regularly, and Dr. Wilson could see the change in her when she went back for her appointment.

"Is the new med helping? Are you getting along better?"

"Yes, I think I am. I am managing daily chores better, but I still wonder when Manny will come back. However, I do get some rest from these thoughts sometimes. Doctor, do you think it is possible that someone could put cameras and microphones in your house to monitor you?"

"Yes, I think it is possible, but I don't think it is at all likely. Do you think someone has done this to you?"

"I had the idea that Manny may have been watching me, but I am not sure now. I haven't heard from him and I thought I would have by now."

"I think that is just a fear you have and you should try to realize that he probably has not done so. What makes you think he did?"

"Well, you know—those round things with the lights that are always on. I think those are cameras."

"What do you mean?"

"They are round and up near the ceiling and my dad says they are 'smoke alarms.'"

"Oh, those. See, we have some here. Look in the corner." The doctor pointed. "All they do is monitor for smoke in case there is a fire."

"Are you sure? Maybe someone is watching you."

"No, I am sure. I have them in my home, too. They are not scary. They're good to have in the house in case a fire breaks out."

"I am not sure. But I will think about it."

"I'm glad that you are feeling better. Keep up the good work and especially keeping taking your meds. You look so much better. I'll see you next month. And Suzy, you need to start thinking about your future."

Suzy's mind was clearer now, and she thought about the smoke alarms. Her parents and sister had them in their homes too. Her sister coaxed her into trying to believe that they weren't cameras. After a week or so, she shyly asked her father to replace the smoke alarms in her house. He was surprised and pleased.

Sometimes at night, she worried about Manny, thinking that he was trying to get in touch with her and not able to for some reason. She still talked about him with anyone who would listen to her, but somehow he wasn't the only important thing in her life. She began to take pleasure in nice weather and good food, and not being miserable about Manny.

~*~

Suzy continued to make slow but steady progress. Then, suddenly, everything changed. Even though she was doing better, she kept a watch on Manny's fan page. She watched his schedule and kept track of when and where he was playing. Even though her obsession had waned, she still found herself unable to stop checking up on him.

One morning, right after breakfast as was her routine, she opened up the fan page to discover that all of Manny's concerts were cancelled. She didn't know what to think. Why would he just cancel everything? She was puzzled and worried. "Manny, she said to herself, "what's wrong? What would keep you from working?"

She didn't even try to get in touch with Trey or any of the band members; she knew that was useless. But she watched the magazines and the tabloids closely. At first, nothing. Not even a whisper of what could be wrong, if anything. She was at the grocery store one evening, doing her weekly shopping. After she loaded her truck with her purchases, she went to the newsstand next door to see if there was any news.

This time she saw a tabloid with a story flagged about him and his "illness." She grabbed the magazine and before even thinking of paying for it, skimmed the story. It was worse than she could have imagined. She staggered against the wall. Finally, she took the magazine up to the cashier, an old man with glasses and a beard.

"Did you see this?" she asked.

The old man, completely disinterested, allowed that he had not. "No, I couldn't possibly read everything that comes through here."

"It's about Emmanuel Sanchez. It says here he has lung cancer and has only a few months to live. You know, he loves me and I love him. He wrote a song for me. He sends me flowers. He can't be dying!"

"I'm sorry to hear that. It'll be $2.50"

Suzy found a five and hastily gave it to him, barely waiting for her change and getting out of there and into her truck and then back home as soon as possible.

Suzy tried phoning but could not get past the gatekeepers. She wrote him letters but got no response. She was so sick over the news that she took to her bed and stopped taking her medication. Her psychosis returned and she thought she was being watched again. Also, her fixation with Manny intensified.

After the news broke, Manny's fan page updated and started letting the fans know how he was without going into detail. Suzy read it avidly, trying to wring as much information as possible out of it. She couldn't believe he was going to die without contacting her. The thought tore at her; she ached to speak with him again. But she heard nothing. Her stomach hurt, and her heart was broken. Manny was the only man she ever really loved and he was dying. She withdrew into herself. All she could think about was Manny and his illness.

She knew the people spying on her had returned, but this time she didn't care. Let them. Let them see how grief-stricken she was, and how much this was hurting her. She didn't care about anything but Manny. She read the messages he left for his fans on his page, trying to grasp any meaning directed at her. A couple of times she was sure he was speaking directly to her, but didn't want anyone to know. She cried, and told him silently that she still loved him. She knew he didn't mean to hurt her; he was just so sick he hadn't had time to get back in touch with her. She was sure he still loved her.

It was agonizing, knowing that he was sick and she couldn't comfort him. Suzy heard about his death on CNN. She cried out, then her face twisted and the tears flowed. How could she live in a world without Manny? She knew he loved her until the end. She told her mother, who came over to check on her and found her bedroom walls covered with pictures of him, "I know he died with my picture in his hand. I am so glad I sent it to him."

Suzy wasn't sure she could stand the pain, but soon found that a person didn't die of pain, and she would have to live with it. After a while, Suzy found herself wanting to die. She always had pills in the house; however, something told her that as hurt as she was over Manny's death, she was young, and she would eventually be able to function again, if she didn't kill herself first. After a few months of struggling between life and death, she went back to her doctor.

Jackie

Chapter Seven

Jackie Renee Allison was tall and had a killer figure. She put on her tight white pants, white halter-top, and sandals adorned with big flowers on the toes. Her parents were babysitting her three-year-old, David, and she felt free as a schoolgirl on Saturday. The bright summer day in Dallas called for sunglasses and she tossed her long blond hair as she put them on. Her brand-new, turquoise and white Thunderbird, a present from her father to help her get over her divorce, glistened as it waited in the driveway, begging to be taken for a spin with the top down, of course.

The wind in her hair felt decadent. She glanced in the mirror to assure herself she looked hot. Impishly, she wondered what it would be like to drive down the wrong way on the one-way street just ahead. Promptly, without thought, she turned the wheel. Nothing happened. She drove back and did it again. And again, faster. The fourth time, driving about thirty miles over the speed limit, she rammed head-on into a delivery truck.

The airbag in Jackie's car went off with a bang! And a poof! Jackie was dazed and so startled she wasn't sure she was all right when she climbed out of the car.

The truck driver hollered, "Lady, are you okay?"

Jackie, with her hands on the back of her head, said quietly, "Yes, I think so."

The truck driver, a big guy with a sweaty t-shirt and long hair, jumped out of the cab and started screaming at her. "What the fuck were you doing, lady? This is a one-way street. I couldn't help hitting you when you came speeding at me. What did you expect me to do?"

Jackie looked at him expectantly. "Look what you've done to my new car. It's ruined. Your company owes me a lot of money, mister. You can't get away with it."

"Shit, I can't believe this! You caused this mess. Why were you driving the wrong way, anyway?"

"I just wanted to see what would happen if I drove the wrong way. You should have seen me coming."

The truck driver shook his head and got back in the truck, calling on his radio, asking the dispatcher to call the police for him, explaining he had a real nut on his hands and needed help with the person who just damaged his truck and messed up his schedule.

Distracted by the people gathering to look at her smashed car, Jackie started to walk away, but a man in a suit grabbed her by the wrist and said, "Oh, no, I saw what happened and you can't just walk away from this. The accident was entirely your fault."

Jackie shook her head, but didn't try to leave again. When the police arrived a few minutes later, the truck driver loudly described the accident backed up by the spectators. Crying, Jackie said she didn't know how she got here or how the accident happened. She was vague and acted lost. The policeman asked Jackie her name, her parents' names, and her telephone number, but she couldn't remember any of this. She noticed he was young, brown-haired, and had the chiseled face she expected a patrolman to sport.

She started shaking while continuing to cry. The policeman was gentle with her, but she wouldn't, or couldn't, tell him anything. Finally, he placed handcuffs on her and put her in the back of the squad car. Her car had already been towed to the impound. She felt small and fettered like a caged finch in the squad car. All the people were looking at her and she had no place to hide. She looked down and let her hair hide her face.

The police radio grumbled and growled incoherently while they went for a long drive out into the country. Jackie didn't know where they were going or why she was being taken away by the cops, and couldn't remember how she got in this predicament. When she wouldn't respond to any questions or attempts at conversation, the officers ignored her and carried on a conversation between themselves, talking about some soccer games; Jackie couldn't make any sense of it.

Finally, they drove up to a big building surrounded by trees. One of the policemen said, cheerily, "Well, here we are." Jackie didn't know where "here" was or what the building was supposed to be. She was lifted out of the car and frog-walked through the entrance.

Inside was a large battered desk with a security guard sitting at the entrance, with a red-haired woman dressed in scrubs. "What have we here?"

The young policeman explained, "This lady had a wreck in town and then couldn't tell us who she was or where she lived. We thought it best to bring her to you guys."

"Okay, we'll find out who she is and contact her relatives. You'll go to court on this?"

"Yes, it should be routine."

"Thanks, guys. See you later."

When the cops left, Jackie felt abandoned. The redheaded woman with freckles splattered on her face like red glitter took Jackie's purse and started going through it, while talking in what the woman probably thought was a soothing manner to Jackie. Jackie's antennae went up and she was ready for anything that might be coming.

The middle-aged security guard with a big belly took her arm and escorted her to another room furnished with a desk and two chairs. Another woman, this one with thin, stringy brown hair, dressed in a suit, asked her the same questions that everyone seemed to be asking

"Name?

"Address?

Telephone number?

Parents' names?"

Jackie wasn't going to talk to this complete stranger. This whole thing was just too much.

Soon, a man, young and with a bad haircut, who had a shaving accident that morning, also dressed in scrubs, came into the room and asked a bunch of questions. Jackie didn't answer, but the woman with red hair gave him Jackie's name, and told him she had spoken with Jackie's parents, and they had given her some information.

"They told me Jackie was newly divorced and was previously mentally ill. They also said her younger brother, Jim, shot himself in the head during halftime while they were all watching last year's Super Bowl. Just excused himself and went out into the garage. No warning. They are extremely worried about Jackie and want us to keep her here while we try to figure out what to do."

The young doctor said, "Oh, I see. Well, let's give her a sedative tonight and see if she feels like talking in the morning. I'm glad you found her relatives. That makes it so much easier. Get her out of those clothes and into a hospital gown and I'll give her a shot."

His statement frightened Jackie even more, but at least she knew what the plan was, so she remained passive while the nurse undressed her and re-dressed her in a gown. The doctor came back in and gave her a shot without saying a word to her.

The nurse with the red hair then led her down a hall to a dingy little room with a bed in it and a small bath off to the side. It had a tiny barred window with cheap-looking curtains.

She tucked Jackie into bed, "Don't be scared, I'll be here to take care of you. Now sleep well and we'll see how you feel in the morning. Good night."

Jackie turned her face to the wall and drifted off into a drug-induced sleep.

Chapter Eight

Jackie woke up with a start in the night. A hand covered her mouth. The pressure on her mouth was unbearable. It was mostly dark, but some light filtered in around the closed door. The silhouette of a big man with a crew cut loomed over her. With one swipe of his hand, he pulled down the sheet covering her, and opened her gown. "Shhh," he hissed, "Don't make a sound."

Terrified, Jackie couldn't remember where she was, but she knew what was coming. In the quiet, she heard the man unzip, then he thrust himself into her. The thrusting felt like a fist jammed inside her. He stiffened. It was over in a minute. Jackie cried quietly in horror.

"Don't tell anyone about this, but it don't really matter because no one will believe you anyhow."

Then he turned and slipped away. Jackie spent the rest of the night crying, this time with her face to the door, waiting and watching for the man to come back. Eventually it was dawn, and a nurse came in to check on her.

Jackie grabbed her sleeve and blurted out, "A man came in here last night and raped me!"

She was sore and tender and knew she was bruised. The nurse, a middle-aged woman with steely-grey hair, pried her fingers from her arm and shushed her. "No, that was just a bad dream. It happens sometimes when it is your first night here and you have been given sleeping drugs. It can be frightening the first night you are here."

"No, no, look at me—I've been raped."

"Now you'll feel better as soon as you've eaten some breakfast and talked to doctor. Just rest now and you'll have something to eat soon. I know it is hard in a strange place."

Jackie realized the man told her the truth; no one here would believe her. She was at his mercy and just had to figure out how to get out of this place as fast as possible. She wondered why the nurse wouldn't believe her.

She had breakfast in a common area with the other patients on the floor. They seemed friendly enough, for the most part. Some of them asked her name, though others didn't talk at all. They gave her nicotine gum when she asked for a cigarette after she ate, which was a sorry substitute for a cigarette but allowed her to hang on to her sanity by her fingernails. Afterwards, they all sat around in the break room with the TV on until it was their turn to talk to the doctor.

When Jackie was called in, a young doctor interviewed her, looking like he just got out of school, just like the one who gave her the shot last night. She thought she would try again, so after he introduced himself as Doctor Casey, she said, "Doctor, a man came into my room last night and raped me. He hurt me so bad and I didn't know what would happen next."

Doctor Casey said, "I'm sorry you had to go through that. It is difficult to adjust to a new place, especially when you have been forced to come here and then are given sleeping medication. I'm sure you'll sleep better as you get used to us."

Staring at him, she didn't know what to say. She was so frustrated, but she told herself, No use trying. He doesn't believe me either. What do I have to do to get someone to believe me?

He started asking her questions such as, "Your birthdate?" Place of birth? Extent of education?"

She answered him, and then he got into the psychological questions. "Does your mind race? Have you lost interest in things you used to enjoy? Are you anxious?"

Jackie found those harder to answer, but Dr. Casey seemed satisfied with her answers. Then he asked her for a narrative of how she got there. By now, Jackie had calmed down and she could remember the events that happened the day before.

At the end of the interview, he said, "I think you have bipolar disorder, and you were having a manic episode when you had your wreck yesterday. I am going to start you on Paxil and Depakote and see how you do. It will take a couple of weeks before you respond to these drugs, so it is a waiting game. Your parents are coming to visit today, so the nurses will give you your makeup from your purse and an opportunity to fix yourself up."

"Oh, thank god. Someone who will listen to me. I have been diagnosed before with depression, but not with bipolar disorder."

"That often happens. You don't get the bipolar diagnosis until mania manifests itself. We are certain it is what you have now, and I'm hoping those are the drugs you respond to. Try to rest today and I will see you tomorrow. Be sure and take your drugs when the nurses ask you to. Goodbye."

Jackie went back to the break room, where she sat down and stared at the muted TV. Soon a small woman with black, curly hair and dark brown eyes sat down beside her and asked, "How are you?"

Jackie started telling her about her car wreck the day before that led up to her ending up in this "institution" as she called it, and soon both of them were giggling. Sarah, as her name turned out to be, had a less funny story to tell. She made it sound funny, describing her husband. "Who up and decided I was crazy as a hooty owl, so he told me, in a soothing voice, almost baby talk, that we were going for a nice drive in the country, When we got here, he gave me the bum's rush, left me at the front desk, and made a run for it."

"Boy, we sure have a way of scaring people, don't we?" said Jackie, laughingly. Then she got serious and told Sarah about the rape she suffered the night before. Sarah said, "I heard about that from someone else, and you know what? The staff never listened to her or believed her. She just had to suck it up."

"Tell me about it. However, my parents are coming to see me this afternoon and I intend to tell them all about it. I think I ought to sue this place for letting it happen to me. They should take better care of patients than that."

"They certainly should. I hope your parents give them what-for. Oh, there's the nurse calling me. It's time for my meds. We're trying something new today. My husband is bringing my little boy to visit and I can't wait to see him. I'll talk to you later."

Jackie felt a little better about being in the hospital after finding someone she could talk to. She hadn't asked the woman what her diagnosis was or how long she had been here, but they could catch up later. It was nice someone finally believed her, too.

She started to cry, thinking of what happened to her the night before and how scary it was. No one paid any attention to her; everyone else was wrapped up in her own problems. She finally sniffled her last, after about half an hour, when the nurse came in and asked her if she wanted her make-up, since her parents would be visiting in about an hour. Jackie said, "Yes," and perked up. At last, she could talk with people who knew her and cared about her.

Chapter Nine

Jackie's name blared through the hospital PA system and she ran out to the lobby to meet her parents. Her father looked the same as always, thin, with skimpy brown hair and eyes that said he wasn't in charge. Her mother's bleached platinum hair was fixed to death—not a strand of it could move, perfectly made up, and with eyebrows that always looked quizzical. They looked like a couple who had stuck together even though it had been rough for them at times.

She wanted to hug both of them long and hard, but they weren't touchy-feely people and couldn't remember the last time they hugged.

"Oh, Mom and Dad, it is so good to see you! It has been a nightmare here. A man sneaked into my room last night and raped me! You need to contact the police for me. The doctors and nurses won't believe me."

"Jackie, that is terrible. How could it happen? Are you all right? We must talk to the doctor about that. I am so sorry. We have to do something about it"

"Mom, I knew you would. Now can you get me out of this place?"

"We need to talk with your doctor first. I think you need to stay here until they can get you stabilized. You are still on Tony's insurance along with David. We didn't bring David with us because we weren't sure what kind of shape you were in and we didn't want to upset him. But he certainly misses his mother. Speaking of that, we have some papers you need to sign for us. They will give us the ability to get medical care for him while you are in the hospital. It's only temporary."

Her mother shoved some legal-looking papers at her. Trusting her parents, Jackie signed the papers without even reading them. She knew her parents needed permission to get medical care for her son. She was grateful to her ex-husband for keeping them both on his hospitalization plan. She wouldn't be getting help without it.

"How are you feeling now?" Her father asked.

"I feel better, but I am still confused and upset. No one will listen to me and I'm so scared. I can't sleep with that man on the loose."

"You must be scared. We can't take you home yet; the doctor says you need to be stabilized first. We will talk to him again. We aren't going to let anything happen to you. Tony's insurance covers two weeks of inpatient care, so you are fine here for a while."

"No, I'm not. It might happen again. Tonight!"

"I told you we will speak to the doctor. Everything will be fine. Now we need to get home to David, but we will make sure you are safe here. Bye, dear."

Jackie went back to the break room feeling a little better. Sarah was there, and Jackie told her about her parents' visit. "Just you wait. The cops will come storming in here in no time," Jackie said. While they waited, they exchanged stories about their children and their plans for the future. Jackie was saddened when Sarah said, "My insurance runs out tomorrow so I won't be able to talk to you anymore. Here, take my phone number for when you get out. We can talk then."

No policemen showed up. Jackie thought that maybe they were there when the nurse called her, but it was only for her second medication dose of the day. When she talked briefly with the doctor, she asked him if her parents had told him about the rape. He just said, "Yes, they told me you mentioned it. But I don't want to upset the staff by making it public." Jackie's mouth dropped open and her heart sank, but she didn't say anything. If they weren't going to do anything about it, she was just going to shut up about it.

When it was time for her to go to bed, she asked the night nurse, a sympathetic-looking fiftyish woman, to leave the light on in her room. The nurse said, "No, you won't be able to sleep that way."

"I won't be able to sleep with it off. Please, please leave it on"

"Okay," said the nurse, "we'll leave it on for a while and see how you sleep. I'll check on you later."

Jackie went to bed as instructed, but was wide-awake. Her heart beat fast and her stomach was roiling. What would she do if the man came back? He was so right that no one believed her. She was at his mercy. Lying with her head turned toward the door, her eyes were wide open for two hours. It was like sleeping on a bed of nails.

Finally, the nurse came in and said, "You aren't going to sleep at all. I've called the doctor to come and give you a sleeping medication and then we can turn off the light."

"No, I'll go to sleep on my own. Just leave the light on and I'll shut my eyes. You'll see."

"One of your problems is you don't sleep enough. That throws you into mania and then the medication can't work for you. We have to make certain you sleep enough. We can't have you lying awake all night."

Just then, a young doctor arrived, one Jackie had not met before. He carried a syringe in his right hand. "Let me give you this and you can go right off to sleep."

"No, please don't give me that. I can sleep by myself."

"We just want to make sure you sleep. Jackie turned away and pulled her arm away from him. "Nurse, hold her arm." Between the two of them, they stretched her arm out straight like a caduceus staff. With that, he injected a liquid into her arm and both he and the nurse pulled the covers up to her neck.

"Nurse, turn out the light and she'll sleep peacefully now."

Jackie lay rigid in the bed, still scared. She decided she would scream as loud as she could if he came back. After a few minutes though, she couldn't keep her eyes open no matter how hard she tried. She wanted to stay awake to try to protect herself, but it was impossible.

When she woke up, the sun was shining into her room and the birds were chirping. The morning nurse bustled into her room to make sure she was awake and tell her it was time to eat.

Jackie was so relieved nothing happened during the night she almost felt good. She was able to eat breakfast and to have a quick conversation with Sarah.

"I'm sorry you have to go now but I promise to call you when I get out. It has been great meeting you and talking with you. It makes me feel like I have a friend."

"You are my friend. We'll catch up when you call me." Sarah hurried off to start the discharge process. Her husband and children were already waiting to pick her up and take her home.

Jackie felt a little more relaxed and was able to think about something other than the rape. She was slowly reconciling herself to the fact nothing was going to be done about it. She questioned herself as to whether she could have imagined it, but she knew she didn't. Jackie knew if any of the doctors or nurses would bother to examine her, they would see the bruises. By now, though, she couldn't show that they happened here. However, not even her parents believed her enough to make a fuss. It made her feel so helpless. She would concentrate on getting better and getting out of this place so it wouldn't happen again.

That was really her only defense, from what she could see. No one was going to take care of her but herself.

Chapter Ten

Dr. Casey checked on her after she had another dose of medication. "My appetite has increased so much that I can't satisfy my hunger, no matter how much I eat. I am hungry between meals and in the night," Jackie complained, "It's distressing and I don't want to get fat."

Dr. Casey replied, "That is a side effect of Depakote. Some people suffer that and you will be uncomfortable and gain a lot of weight if you continue taking it. Don't worry, I'll change your medication to Risperdal. It doesn't have that side effect, and we will see how that works. Your mania has receded and you can go home as soon as you feel strong enough. We'll refer you to a psychiatrist in the community who will follow up on your care. Do you have a place to live?"

"I have been living with my parents since my divorce. I guess I will go back there. They have been caring for my son since I have been here, and I miss him. I can't wait to see him."

"Talk with your parents about when you can return home. I'll sign you out when they are ready. They will be here later today, they told me."

"Okay."

Jackie settled herself in the break room to wait. It was a little room with four or five scarred blonde tables and chairs scattered around the room. There were games and cards spread around. In one corner, there was a TV with rabbit ears, but it was usually muted. The facility didn't have cable, so the only thing on were game shows and soap operas. She missed Sarah, but didn't feel like striking up a conversation with anyone else. She was concentrating on getting out of the hospital. Her parents were afraid of mental illness since Jim shot himself, so she would have to keep herself together. It didn't matter how crazy she felt, she would have to act sane when they got there.

She deliberately calmed herself and thought about David and getting to see him. She missed him so much. It had only been a couple of days but she couldn't bear being separated from him any longer. She also didn't want to spend the night in this place again. Jackie always told David, "We are like peas and crackers." It didn't make any sense, but it was funny. He always laughed when she said that. After a while, she was called for Visitors. She went to the lobby and found her mother and father there. She wanted to run up to them, throw her arms around them, and beg them to take her home with them, but she knew how her mother thought. Instead, she walked up to them demurely and asked, "How are you, Mom and Dad?"

They exchanged a glance and her mother said, "We are just fine, dear, and so is David. We wanted to know how you are."

"I'm feeling good and the doctor said my mania is receding. He said I could go home today."

"Are you sure you are ready for that? The doctor told us he gave you a new medication today. Perhaps you should see how that works first."

"Oh, no, I'm sure it will be fine. They will give me the name of a doctor to go to if anything goes wrong and for follow-up."

"Well, I'm not sure, dear. What about you thinking you were raped the first night you were here?"

"I'm sure that was just the effect of the combination of the mania, the drugs, and the fear of being in a strange place. It was all so scary."

Well, your father and I will talk it over. Give us a few minutes."

Jackie went back to the break room, thinking she was not going home today. She started to cry, but then stopped herself through sheer force of will. She wasn't going to screw up her chances now. When her parents called her back into the visitors' room to talk with her again, her mother looked stern and her father uncertain.

Her mother said, "Jackie, we aren't ready to take you home yet. We talked to the doctor and he said you are much better, but he doesn't mind observing you for another day. Tony's insurance will pay for it, and it will give you a better opportunity to get used to your medication. But if everything goes all right, we will take you home tomorrow evening."

Jackie's stomach knotted when she heard she had to spend another night in that horrible little room and she swallowed hard finding out she had wait to see David, but she smiled at her parents, "I'll be ready tomorrow; can't wait to see David. Thanks for all your help. Good night."

Jackie went back to the break room and sobbed. She stayed there until the nurse came to get her to go to bed. This time Jackie pretended to sleep even though it was difficult, and sometime in the middle of the night she did drift off, with thoughts of David soothing her.

The next morning Jackie felt calmer, and she had a purpose. She was going to convince everyone that she was ready to get out of the hospital. She was polite to the nurses and the kitchen staff, and took her medicine graciously. When she talked to Dr. Casey, he told her he assumed she was being discharged and gave her the name, address, and phone number of a psychiatrist close to her parent's home who could follow her care.

"Thank you so much for this. I'm sure he will take good care of me and that I won't get manic like that again. I am really looking forward to seeing my son and I hope you discharge me today," Jackie said.

"I can tell you feel much better. You must take your medicine every day, even when you feel fine, and you have to keep your appointments with the doctor. Bipolar disorder is a lifelong disease. There is no cure, but it can be kept under control if you are vigilant," Dr. Casey replied.

"Yes, doctor, I understand. I'll take care of it and of myself."

Jackie went back to her room and packed up what little she had to go home. The nurses had given her purse, make-up, and clothes back to her, so she was able to get dressed. She waited impatiently, all day, for her parents. When they finally arrived, after supper, the discharge procedure was finished and she was ready to go. Jackie said "good-bye" to Dr. Casey and her nurse and left.

In the car on the way home, her parents tried to make small talk with her, but it was obvious they were apprehensive about taking her home. Jackie didn't feel like she had to pretend anymore; all she cared about was seeing David. She answered questions with grunts and "Mmhms" and looked out the window. She watched the telephone poles go by silently, with their wires sagging and the birds roosting forlornly on them. She was grateful to her parents for getting her out of the hospital, but she was angry that they didn't believe her when she told them she was raped. Nothing would ever make up for that.

Chapter Eleven

When they got home, Jackie rushed inside to see David. Unfortunately, the babysitter already put him to bed and he was asleep. Jackie hesitated for a moment, then ran to his room and woke him up to say "hello" and "I love you."

David was groggy and sleepy, but happy to see his mother, "I love you, too, Mommy," he said, before falling back to sleep. He was a sturdy little boy, with Jackie's blonde hair and his dad's brown eyes. Jackie slept in the same room, so she quietly disrobed and got into bed. It was heaven sleeping in her own bed and feeling safe for the first time since she went to the hospital. She fell asleep immediately and slept all night.

The next morning, Jackie shuffled out to the kitchen in her robe and slippers where her mother made her breakfast. David had already eaten, but sat with Jackie, happy to be near her. Her mother placed her morning pills next to her plate. Jackie had forgotten about them, but took them without question. After the meal, she made for the living room couch and turned on the TV, spending the rest of the day on the couch, staring at the TV. This became her daily routine. David took his naps on the couch with her and turned to her for comfort when his grandmother chided him.

Jackie's mother tried to interest her in activities, but Jackie would not pay any attention to her. She took her meds as long as her mom reminded her. She didn't want to think about anything, especially her time at the hospital.

After the first month, her mother said, "Tomorrow is your first appointment with Dr. Burkhalter, so you will need to get up early and get dressed. You have to be there at ten."

"Oh no," Jackie groaned. "I forgot about that. I'll set the alarm tonight."

The next morning, when the alarm blared, Jackie rolled over with the pillow around her ears until she remembered she had to go to the doctor. She dressed carefully and ate breakfast; then her mother, David, and she got into the car and drove to the office. When she met Dr. Burkhalter, she was impressed by his dignified look and his warmth.

Her mother wanted to come into the appointment with her, but Jackie vetoed that. Her mother managed to get the doctor to promise to talk with her after the meeting with Jackie.

"Jackie, I understand you were in the hospital last month. How do you feel now?"

"I feel fine, Doctor, just a little tired, sometimes."

"Are you taking your medications?"

"Certainly, every day."

"Any problems with your meds?"

"No, not at all."

"Good, just make sure you continue taking them." You must keep that up, or you will never be able to function again. Have you thought about what you are going to do?'

"No, I just went through a divorce and then went to the hospital, so I haven't had much time for thinking."

"You need to make a plan and stick with it. I'll see you again in a month. Take your meds and try to think of what you would like to do with the rest of your life."

"Okay."

When Jackie got home, she took off her clothes and lay down on the couch. There she stayed. Two days later, her mother took a phone call, and came to talk with Jackie.

"That was Tony calling."

"What did that idiot want?"

"He says he has cut off your health insurance because he is afraid your going to the mental hospital will make him look bad. You have one more month of coverage, then nothing. What will you do?"

"I don't know, Mom, but something will work out."

~ * ~

A month later, Jackie got off the couch again to go to Dr. Burkhalter's. This time they went through the regular questions, and then Jackie told him about losing her insurance. "What am I going to do? I won't be able to see you or buy my meds."

"Don't worry; you can go to the Mental Health Clinic. They will see you and help you with your medications. I will give you a referral and you can make an appointment. I'm sorry, though, that you lost your insurance. It's always easier to take care of things when you have insurance. Now have you thought any about what you want to do in the future?"

"I've thought about it, but I haven't come up with anything. I'll keep working on it."

Jackie had only been taking her meds because her mother reminded her. A week after she got home this time, she was lying on the couch watching TV when a show about bipolar disorder came on. It was on "Oprah" and it made Jackie think for the first time in a long time. She learned more about the disorder than she learned at the hospital and from the doctors. Suddenly, she remembered Sarah and her promise to call her.

She retrieved her purse from the bedroom and found the crumpled-up note with the phone number. Fingers shaking, she dialed the number. What she got though, was a recording, saying, "The number you have reached in not in service." Jackie slammed the phone down and then dialed more slowly. Again, she got the recording. She was so angry with herself for forgetting Sarah and she cried a little for missing her chance to be a friend with her. She wondered how she was now.

Jackie went back to her spot on the couch, promising herself she would think about the future.

Missy

Chapter Twelve

Hair tousled, makeup smeared across her face, Melissa Ann Brooks slept so hard it took several minutes for the pounding on her door to register. When she did wake, it was a while before she found her robe amidst the piles of discarded clothes heaped on the floor and chairs. Empty and half-full fast-food containers were on every flat surface, CDs strewn about, and the muted TV flickered in the darkened room. The knocking went on relentlessly. She opened the door; a huge sheriff's deputy stood there. His leather jacket and a brown uniform filled the doorway and a big mustache sprouted from under his nose. It didn't seem to register with him that she was delicate-looking, with shoulder-length black hair and black eyes. She gave him a smile, usually that caused a softening of manner with a man, but there was no response from him, even though when fixed up rather than awakened when she was hung over, she was a knockout.

"Oh, not again!" she exclaimed. Still groggy and unsteady on her feet, but realizing what he was here for. "Oh god. I don't have any money; do what you have to do."

The other two times Missy had been evicted, calling friends, they gathered up her belongings and found another apartment. She charmed the landlords and moved in before they could check her credit. This time she knew she wouldn't be able to find anyone who would be willing to help again. No money for a deposit on a new place, and her car was gone, too, repossessed two weeks ago.

Missy had downed her last bottle of vodka. She was done, no longer feeling capable of taking on the world and winning. Worn out, it was time to call her mother on the cell phone she managed to keep alive and asked her to pick her up. While waiting, she gathered up her makeup and some of her favorite clothing, dodging the men who were arranging her furniture and other possessions next to the curb. This time, Missy didn't even watch them go. She was tired of fighting life in general and ready to give up. She didn't even curse the men when they took her bed, a hard-earned and cherished possession. Giving up, she was standing quietly in front of the apartment with her bags packed next to a pile of clothing with her cat, Stradivarius, in his carrier, waiting for her mother to rescue her.

Her mother finally drove up. Missy expected her to be upset and ready to scold her a mile a minute, but instead her mother gently asked, "Are you going to move in with me this time?"

"Yes, please," Missy said and they drove home in silence. This ended a several-month crazy time in Missy's life.

Six months ago, everything was normal. Missy worked as an automobile insurance agent, had a paid-for car, a nice apartment, a cat, and dated occasionally. Then, her life changed. She found herself attracted to guy she met at a party, Gunther, who was tall and thin, with a pencil-thin mustache and eyes that danced with fun. They started going to a bar several nights a week. He worked part-time, picking up shifts at the Chevrolet plant in Arlington, about thirty miles away from where he lived in Dallas. She drank more and more each night, until consuming a bottle of vodka each time they had a date was normal. Gunther encouraged her to have a good time.

Her work suffered, but she managed to make it to the sparse office often enough to keep it going. She and Gunther had a stormy relationship, but he pledged his undying love for her, and she certainly loved him. While they were out, he would say, "I see you looking at that guy over there."

Missy would reply, "What guy?"

"The one you are making eyes with."

"Gunther, I'm not looking at anyone."

"Yes, you are, and I am going to leave you alone with him."

"Gunther, don't go. I love you and only you. Please take me home and I'll prove it to you."

"No, I'm leaving."

And he would leave. She would sit there, all alone, for a couple of hours, until he cooled off and came back. Then they would go home and make up. They were inseparable, except when one of them got their feelings hurt. They went everywhere together—to the movies, out to eat, to the bar, and they slept every night at either her place or his. Sometimes they fought, but the makeup sex was delicious, and their breakups never lasted more than a few hours.

Gunther, who used Missy's car when he wanted to go out without her, told her she should be ashamed to drive that old, paid-for clunker. "You need something new, bright and shiny, something that sends a message."

Missy hadn't thought about it, but when she looked around, she noted that all of Gunther's friends had brand-new cars, and they did look a lot better than her car. "You're right, Gunther, let's start looking for a new car. It'll be fun."

They went to the car dealerships along Highway 635, in North Dallas, where the dealers were lined up for miles, and must have looked at dozens of cars. As they looked, Missy got an idea of what Gunther wanted. He wanted a red car, a big car, a car with a name that sounded like a man's car. They finally showed up at Montfort Motors, an upscale dealership with music playing on the loudspeakers, free Texas barbeque, and a salesman who kept rubbing his hands while he tried to listen and simultaneously talk to them about buying a car. Missy had made up her mind. She went straight to the car she wanted -- a bright apple-colored Dodge Durango. She teased the salesman a little bit by pretending she was still not quite ready to buy, then broke down and negotiated a price. Gunther was delighted. Missy was so happy that he was happy she didn't worry a bit about the car payment.

Missy paid less and less attention to her job, even though it used to be the most important thing in her life, and her income started to drop off. She made the car payment first and the rent second, and sometimes not at all. It got to be standard that the car was more important than the apartment payment. Still, she was absolutely astonished when she came home at 2 a.m. and found her belongings out by the street and a new lock on the apartment door. She had just ignored the warnings and assumed nothing would happen. In her state of mind, there were no consequences. You just lived your life and everything would work out.

The manager was a soft touch for animals and kept Strad in the office for her. "Gunther, call your friends and get as many of them here as you can. I'll stay here and guard the stuff while you gather up all the people you know with pick-ups." Gunther's friends packed up their cars and trucks with Missy's furniture and belongings. While they did that, Missy went to a complex where she knew the manager. "Listen, I just had this big fight with my manager and we both decided I didn't want to live in her complex anymore. Help me out by letting me move in here. Don't call her; I don't want you involved in her nastiness. She didn't think I should be dating the guy I am dating and let's just leave it at that."

By evening, she was moved in. It was pure luck and nerve. Things did work out. She went clubbing with Gunther every night, drank a whole bottle of vodka, and stayed up all night with him, passed out in the early mornings, seldom made it to work and stopped worrying about anything. As her customers caught on, they deserted her. The insurance company fired her.

On a Saturday night Missy offered to drive one of Gunther's friend's home, because she was sure he was too drunk to drive. "I'll drive you home, and Gunther can follow in my car and take me home after we get to your place." They made it to the first intersection. The deputy who pulled her over didn't fall for her innocent act.

"Officer, I only had two beers tonight."

"I'm going to let you prove that by having you blow into this breathalyzer."

"You'll see I'm not at all drunk."

Missy blew, and blew double the legal limit. She was taken to jail, but when her bail for DWI was set, she couldn't locate Gunther to come and get her.

Chapter Thirteen

"You don't have to do that," she ranted. "I'm not going anywhere. And I'll see you in court and prove to you that I am not drunk." Missy was angry the cop thought she was drunk. She was particularly angry that he insisted on putting handcuffs on her.

Her wrists hurt and she asked, "Can't you take these handcuffs off? You know I am not going to hurt you."

The policeman answered, "It's just policy, ma'am."

"Who are you calling 'ma'am'? My name is Ms. Brooks, I'll have you know."

"Yes, ma'am."

"Oooh" Missy breathed in frustration, but decided not to pursue it. They went to the jail with Missy sitting in the back, one leg swinging. "How come you don't have a partner? You know I could accuse you of rape."

"You could, but I wouldn't advise it, unless you want to go to Parkland and have a rape kit done."

"You think you are pretty smart, don't you?"

When they got to the jail, she was patted down just as she had been when she was standing by the car, and had to answer a bunch of questions as they booked her. They took a lot of her information off her drivers' license, and gave her another breathalyzer test, which infuriated her.

"Why do I have to take another test? I'll sue you for this. This is an invasion of my privacy. I want you to know that I object strenuously to this."

The woman clerk said, "I know you do, but this one's for medical reasons, and I have to give it to you."

She turned her over to another clerk, who finally took off the handcuffs and started to fingerprint her. Now Missy, through a haze, realized that she was actually going to jail and started to cry. She cried while putting on the jail suit, the ugliest thing she ever wore, a white overall with Dallas County Jail in big letters on it. She continued to cry while they put her in a cell with about ten other women.

At first, she just sat on a bench, but after a while, one of the women came and sat beside her and started to talk to her. Missy's curiosity overcame her, and she started asking questions. She found that she didn't have a lot in common with the other women in jail, except for the two who also had DWIs. One of them was passed out and the other one was as angry as Missy was. They traded stories and that helped Missy to calm down.

"I was just driving down the road, minding my own business, and this policeman stopped me for absolutely no reason, accused me of being drunk, and brought me to jail," said the woman.

"That's exactly the same thing that happened to me. What is with these cops? I can't wait to see the judge," Missy responded.

Most of the other women were drunks and a handful were prostitutes. One young woman sat in the corner with her back turned to the others in a deep drug haze. Missy was polite to all of them, and finally asked the friendliest one, "Now how do I get out of here?"

Esther, one of the prostitutes, said, "You'll go to court in the morning, and the judge will set bail. Depending on how many times you have been arrested and whether you live in town and have connections here, such as family, bail will be high or low. Then someone can pay a bail bondsman ten percent of that to get you out."

Missy got one of the guards to take her to the phone. Missy called her mother and told her what happened. She asked her to bail her out in the morning if Gunther couldn't be reached. Her mother was not happy, but promised to come and get her after bond was set if needed. Missy tried several times to reach Gunther earlier, but she couldn't locate him.

When bail was finally set, Gunther still couldn't be reached, so she had to call her mother to pick her up. All the way, home her mother, Susan, bitched at her. "I told you that black boyfriend of yours would do you no good. He's useless—won't even bail you out of jail. What are you doing, drinking so much you get a DWI? Why was he letting you drive? And where is he? Missy, you had better break up with him for good if you don't want to get into even more trouble. I won't be the one to take care of you if you do."

Missy just stared out the window at the bare trees swaying in the cold wind. She said nothing to her mother, but wondered where Gunther was and what he was doing. She couldn't wait to see him. Even though not too happy with him, she knew he had a good excuse for not being Johnny on the spot when needed. If he could have, she knew he would have been there.

It took her two days to locate Gunther at his place, and he apologized profusely for not being around when she needed him. "My mom was sick," he said, "and I had to get her medicine and take her to and from the doctor. Otherwise, you know I would have been right there for you. I am so sorry you had to get your mother to help. I wouldn't have done that to you if there were any way I could have helped it."

"Gunther, is your mother okay? I tried calling you there but no one was home."

"Oh yeah, she's fine now. That's why I'm back at my place now. I wasn't sure where you were, but I knew you would find me here."

"I need you to bring my car over here. My rent is days late and I have saved the money to pay it, but I'm not sure the landlady will accept it now. Please hurry."

"I'll get there as fast as I can but you know I have things to do."

Missy waited impatiently for Gunther, but he didn't show up. She kept trying to reach him by phone, but again, was not able to locate him. Finally, around ten o'clock the next morning, he pulled up in her car. She was more than ready to get to her apartment, so thanked her mother perfunctorily for picking her up and headed out the door. They had spoken little to each other the past few days. Her mother said, "Missy, I don't like the way you are acting, and you are simply throwing your life away on that Gunther."

Missy answered, "You don't understand how I feel about Gunther."

Gunther drove her to her apartment; this time she was not surprised to see her belongings set in the parking lot beside the street. Much of her stuff was missing. Again, since the manager was a friend, she had kept Strad for her. Missy felt a pang of guilt. If not for luck, Strad would be at the pound, maybe dead by now.

Again, Gunther called his friends and this time two of them, who lived in an apartment complex in which most of the tenants were black, vouched for her to the manager and she got an apartment there the same day. She moved but this time she had lost a lot of her belongings. At least she had the basics—no one had hauled off the bigger things, like her bed or dresser.

To Missy, it was just a slight hiccup. She still had Gunther and still partied hearty. Reality didn't really impinge on her life. She no longer went to work at all and her little income came from Gunther. He kept her in alcohol and paid for her cell phone. She no longer paid rent or car insurance or made car payments. None of that seemed important anymore. The only important things were going to the clubs and making love to Gunther every chance she got. No longer in communication with her mother, she knew Susan would bitch at her. Missy just let it go.

Missy was incredibly happy. She gave no thought to the consequences of her actions, and, if she did, they were dismissed immediately. Eviction, hangovers, loss of her business, DWI, nothing seemed real to her. Reality was partying and loving Gunther. At the same time, any little thing could set her off. "Godamnit! How did you get this job?" she screamed at a waiter who got her order wrong.

Or to a grocery clerk, she said, "What is this? Trainee's day? God, you are so slow."

The tiniest things could push her buttons if someone didn't do something the way she wanted them, she became insulting and profane, and was not embarrassed about it all, even later. People should just know how to act.

Sex with Gunther was great, and she craved it all the time. Sometimes, when he wasn't there when she wanted him, it was tempting to call one of his friends to play around with. She didn't, but could have. Missy would lie there and fantasize about it, terribly impatient about Gunther's absence.

She was at his place when a woman came by, all in a snit. "Gunther, you no-account bastard, you haven't bought any diapers or baby formula for Rayna in a month! How do you expect me to make it on my own? I need you to help me."

Missy was right there, in her face, "Who are you? Why are you asking Gunther for help?"

"Because I'm Gunther's baby-mama, that's why. I need help with this baby."

Gunther stepped in front of Missy, opened his wallet, and handed some bills to her. He said, "Belinda, I'll send you some more after I get paid next week."

"Is this white woman keeping you from paying me? Are you spending so much on her that you haven't got money for your own children?"

"No, Belinda, I just haven't seen you in a while and I forgot."

"Well, you better be sending some cash to Bertha, too, because she's looking for you."

"Okay, I will. Leave, I will come over and see you and Reyna later."

"You better. And you, if you have any sense, you'll stay away from this one."

Belinda turned her back and left.

Missy blew up like Mount St. Helen's. "What is this about a baby-mama?" she ranted. "Two baby-mamas? Gunther, you never told me about this. How dare you keep these secrets from me!"

"I knew you wouldn't take it well, that's why I didn't tell you. After all, it's really none of your business."

"None of my business?" said Missy. "You have two children and it is none of my business? We'll see about that."

Missy was angry, to say the least. She was also hurt and crying, in that unattractive, air gasping, sobbing way.

When an unfazed Gunther just looked at her, she turned her back and stormed out of the apartment.

Chapter Fourteen

Missy drove around aimlessly, alternately weeping and pounding the steering wheel. She was talking to herself, "Why did I fall for his shit; I will never let him touch me again, no matter what." After a couple of hours, the drive calmed her enough that she went home. The first thing she did was to block his phone number and the second was to call a locksmith to change the lock, not telling the manager because the rent hadn't been paid and she didn't think it would be a good idea. The last thing she did was to park her Durango in the parking lot next door, so Gunther wouldn't find it.

She drank and cried all night. Finally, toward morning, sleep came. When she woke up, it was almost time to go to the club. She fixed herself up, more carefully than had been her habit in recent weeks, and sailed out the door. Missy stopped at an auto parts store on the way and bought steering wheel lock, because she assumed Gunther had made a key for the car. She wouldn't put anything past him.

As soon as she walked into the dark, mirrored bar, Gunther eased up to her. "Missy, I have been waiting for you. We need to talk." Missy pushed by him and went to the bar to order a drink. Gunther followed her.

"Missy, those girls have nothing to do with our lives. Everything is over between them and me. It's just that they have my kids and…"

Missy ostentatiously ignored him, She stepped in between two of his friends, "Hi, How are you guys tonight?"

They looked at her warily. "Fine, fine. Aren't you with Gunther?"

"No, not anymore."

"Well, you'll make up."

"Not this time."

They moved away from her. She spent the evening going from group to group, finally finding Jimmy who agreed to go to her house.

"Hey, Jimmy, I've had fun tonight. Would you like to come home with me and have some coffee?"

After they got to her place, sex with Jimmy felt good. It helped cut the ties to Gunther. From then on, Gunther did not speak with her and she had a new man every night. For some reason, Missy didn't feel as good as before, but kept trying to get the feeling back. After a couple of weeks or so, she woke up on a Wednesday and when she went outside to start to run errands, her car was not where she parked it.

"Damn that Gunther! I knew he would do this," she exclaimed. She hadn't bothered with the steering wheel lock the past few days since he was studiously ignoring her.

She grabbed up her phone, shaking with anger. She punched in "911" and when the operator said "911, what is your emergency?" Missy said, "Someone stole my car and I can even tell you who it was."

The operator said, "What is the license number of the car?"

"Why do you need to know that? I know who stole it."

"Please give me the license number."

Missy, angry, spat out the license number to her and the operator said, "One moment, please."

Missy couldn't believe she was sitting on hold on 911. She had a real emergency here and the operator wasn't listening to her. No telling what Gunther would do to her car if they didn't catch up to him soon. She was seething. The operator came back on the line. "What were you doing? I need help here."

"I'm sorry, ma'am, I was just checking the database. Your car, which is a red Dodge Durango, right?"

"Yes, it is. I could have told you that."

"Has not been stolen, it was repossessed this morning at nine a.m."

"Oh shit!" Missy hung up.

From then on, Missy had to get rides to the club and to the store and wherever else she had to go. It wasn't difficult, but it was a pain to have to wait on someone else to get things done.

"Jimmy, before you leave this morning, could you give me a ride to the supermarket? I need to get some groceries," asked Missy in a phone call.

"No, I need to get to work. Sorry, got to go now."

Missy called around until she found someone who would help. She still didn't feel like calling her mother. Not wanting to hear "I told you so," even knowing her mother would be justified in everything she said. Missy just wasn't up to it. If the truth were known, she could use a mother's comfort right now. Life had let her down, nothing she did was right; everything had crumbled on her. She felt like an abandoned child. Picking up men at the club wasn't fun anymore.

One night she came home earlier than usual. The guy just dropped her off because she didn't even feel like having sex. Missy desultorily watched TV and petted Strad. Finally, she went to bed alone and depressed. The next morning, persistent banging on her door woke her. The sheriff had found her at home this time.

Chapter Fifteen

Her mother's old and outdated furniture sparkled in the clean and perfectly neat house. Missy was small when her father left Susan, her mother, to care for their daughter as a single mom. When they both arrived home, she showed Strad where the food bowl and the litter box were. Then Missy put some sheets on the bed in the guest bedroom. Without even undressing, she dropped onto the bed and was immediately asleep.

Missy woke up at 4:00 p.m. with her mother waiting for her with dinner, and she wanted to talk.

"Missy, I need to know what has been going on these past few months."

Missy gave her a sanitized version of what had happened. Even cleaned up, it was pretty awful. Her mother didn't say, "I told you so," but her tone did when she spoke. Susan was small and slight, and her dark hair was shot with grey. Missy got her features from her. Still an attractive woman, but obviously over fifty, she looked sad and put-upon.

"Missy do these things you've told me sound right to you?" her mother asked.

"No," Missy said, 'I don't know why I was doing the things I was. It doesn't even seem like me."

"Your aunt, Blanche, who died before you ever knew her, used to do strange things like that, and I think she was mentally ill. I believe you should get some help from the Mental Health Center."

"Me? Mentally ill? Don't be ridiculous. I'm not crazy."

"Maybe not, but think about it. I don't want to see you go through this again. Anyway, from now on I'm going to wake you when I leave for work. I know your schedule is all messed up, but I expect you to get up. By Friday, you will have dinner on the table when I get home. Also, I expect you to take over all the care for all the cats, not just yours, but my two also. And spend some time thinking about what I said about Blanche."

Susan went to bed and of course, Missy wasn't tired. She found a jigsaw puzzle and worked it until 5:00 a.m. By then she felt sleepy and went to bed. At 7:00, her mother woke her up and made her eat Kashi cereal and have some coffee. As soon as her mother left, Missy went back to bed. However, this time she woke at 2:30 p.m. and each day she went to bed earlier and got up earlier until she was able to cook supper.

On Saturday, Missy, who was subdued now, helped her mother with the cleaning. Then, as they sat in the kitchen, said, "Mom, tell me more about Aunt Blanche."

"I never talk about her much because it is so sad. Blanche did well in school, and married right after high school. She had two children right away. Suddenly she started to ignore the children and stay out all night. Her husband was beside himself. He had to work and take care of the kids—he didn't know where Blanche was half the time. But he loved her. Just about the time he was going to file for divorce, she came home and begged him to forgive her. Said she didn't know what came over her and that it would never happen again.

Everything was fine for a while. Then, in about two years, the same thing happened. This time Robert divorced her, got full custody of the children, and moved to California. We never heard from them again. Blanche was heartbroken when she came to her senses. She got married two more times, but the same thing kept happening. What you have gone through has reminded me of Blanche. She killed herself, Missy."

"Oh my god. You never told me any of this. How did she do it?"

"She hanged herself in her closet. I didn't want to tell you. I hoped it was Blanche's problem and it would never happen again. But Missy, I think you're acting just like her. Please think about getting some treatment. I don't know what was wrong with Blanche, but they know so much more about these things than they used to."

"But, Mom, I'm not crazy. I always know what I am doing."

"Maybe so, but think about Blanche. She ruined her life, and made herself so unhappy she killed herself."

Melissa thought about what her mother told her for about two weeks, and finally decided it wouldn't hurt her to talk with a therapist of some kind. She couldn't get her aunt's suicide out of her mind, and called the Mental Health Clinic for an appointment. The earliest one she could get was in three weeks.

~ * ~

When she got to her appointment at the Mental Health Clinic, rather a dreary place, she was surprised to see that her doctor was a woman, Dr. Hettinger. The doctor asked her why she had come in, and Missy told her about last summer and how weird it had all been. The doctor asked her a few more questions, then,

"Missy, I think you have a classic manic condition, bipolar disorder, which means you lose control of your moods. Your moods go up and down without your input. You are a Type I, which means you lean more to the manic side of the illness, and you have less depression. The disease is cyclical, so unless you take medication, you will suffer for the rest of your life."

"But I can take medication and stop it?"

"We can usually find appropriate medication that will break the cycle and allow you to live a normal life. But be prepared, it can take a long time to find the right medication for you. If we are lucky, we will find it right away, if not, it may take several tries to get it right."

"What do I have to do?"

"Just take the medications I prescribe. Let me know if you have any side effects and it really helps if you keep a mood chart, that is, keep track of any fluctuations in your mood, just to be conscious of your moods."

"It sounds like a fulltime job."

"It practically is, at first. Once we have your medications right, you can go several months without seeing a doctor and just take your meds every day. It's not so bad then."

"Oh, okay. Well, let's get started."

Marie

Chapter Sixteen

Opal Marie White slammed on the brakes just before rear-ending the green Chrysler in front of her. Busy trying to figure out where she was, she didn't see the light change. Close to tears, frustrated, she raised her voice and let out some unladylike curses. When she was moving to Dallas two weeks ago, Marie didn't consider the part about having to learn a whole new town layout. She lived in Oklahoma City most of her life and could get around there on instinct.

As she explained to her sister, Shirley, living in Oklahoma City had lost its attractiveness. "With all this bad stuff happening I just feel like I have to get out of here." First, Brad died of that sudden heart attack. That was a shock, he wasn't that old. She didn't have any plans for that.

After Marie made it through Brad's funeral, comforting his son, Ben, as much as she could, she had a meeting with their lawyer. Josh was always one of her favorite friends. He was soft-spoken and gentle, got along great with kids, and was honest almost to a fault Marie was expecting their meeting to be routine.

Josh, tall and lanky, greeted her and said, "Marie, I am so sorry about Brad's death. I know you will miss him. You two had such a wonderful marriage but it ended too soon. I wish I were here to give you good news."

Marie, startled, felt a small ball of fear in her stomach. Her palms started to sweat. What did he mean? "Marie, this will be a shock for you, but Brad left all his money in trust for Ben. I doubt you expected anything like that, but he seemed to think you could take care of yourself while Ben needed money to go to college and he wanted the best for him."

"How could he do that?" demanded Marie. "I expected to be in good shape financially. This is awful." Nervously, Marie began to twist a hank of her hair through her fingers.

"That isn't all," Josh went on, "Brad left you half the house, the other half to Ben, and so you have to sell it. That's all the money you get from the estate. I'm sorry, Marie."

"It's not your fault, Josh. But it is a huge surprise, I am still working at MedPrime, so it will be all right. I just need some time to adjust."

Marie had been with MedPrime as a medical writer for nine years, and believed she could work there until retirement. She was happy in her job and knew they were happy with her. True, she was angry with Brad, but the situation wasn't dire. She had trouble holding onto a job before she found the right meds for her bipolar disorder, but had done fine since then.

After Brad's death and her surprise about the money, things started going south. A person would never know Marie had bipolar disorder just by looking at or talking with her. She was on the same medications for twelve years and they had kept her stable. Now, the medications failed her. She developed an allergy to it. Her regular doctor seemed at a loss as to what to do. "Stop taking the medication, he said, and go to the pharmacy for some skin cream."

That didn't seem like much of a plan to Marie. Desperate, dragging out the Yellow Pages and looking up "Psychiatrists," Marie found the nearest one. She knew it was not a scientific way to find a good doctor, but it was her preferred method. She called, and made an appointment for the next week, trying to stay on an even keel at work.

At the first appointment with the new doctor, Dr. Molina, she had to explain the long road that got her to his office. Marie explained she had bipolar disorder and had taken medication for it for nearly twelve years. "This kept me from holding a steady job for most of my working life. I tried several careers, worked as a social worker, a teacher, a paralegal, and at last getting the position I wanted, as a writer. I have worked as a medical writer for nine years, and it is my dream job."

"I am happy at MedPrime, and after only three years I was given a promotion and a substantial raise. After all the failures I racked up, this was a real shift. It was nice to be valued; all this had come after my diagnosis and getting on the right medications."

"Years ago," she explained, "I was finally diagnosed of cycling from mania to depression every few months, but after that I spent five years trying to find the correct medication to stabilize my illness. I took the lithium prescribed for me, but it had no effect. The doctors told me, 'That's impossible. The med is working for you, you just can't tell it'."

"As a last resort, I checked into a hospital and got the right med. At the hospital, the resident said, 'You don't need to take lithium because it is not working for you. I'm going to try you on a new medication'."

"I tried what he prescribed, and became stable in a week, to my great relief. I felt that the resident had saved my life. I was so unhappy living with the disorder, knowing it could be controlled, but I was not making any progress toward managing it before I got on the proper meds."

Dr. Molina said, "It can be difficult to find the appropriate medication, and that was especially true fifteen years ago."

"Dr. Molina, those weren't my only problems. I had trouble with relationships, too. After some really bad ones,

[85]

I vowed never to marry, knowing it would not work. This seemed particularly true after spending ten years in love with Ted, who obviously did not love me back and finally left me with no warning. It must be a bipolar thing. Who would stay in love with a man who didn't love her back for ten years? It took me a long time to get over that. That was followed by several subsequent, shorter bad relationships, until I was diagnosed, and, again, was put on the proper medication."

"When I met Brad, he said 'I know all about bipolar disorder and it doesn't bother me.' We had a good, healthy relationship and within a year, he overcame my fears and asked me to marry him. He understood my limitations and ours was a happy marriage, but all too short."

The most distressing part of my situation is I just got a new RN for a supervisor and my old boss was promoted. I don't know the new supervisor well; I am lead writer for my group and have basically been heading it up for months. The new boss started by saying, 'I am sure you will resent having a boss after all this time of supervising your workers.'

'No, I am glad to have a supervisor to take some of the administrative work off me. I welcome your help,' I answered. Ellen, the new RN, did not seem to believe me. I have been trying to keep up appearances and hoping I could pull it off until a new medication is effective."

Dr. Molina responded, "I just heard about a new medication that is supposed to be really effective. I'll start you on it immediately and I hope you can get back up to speed in a few weeks."

At her next appointment Marie said, "I've been depressed and I haven't been sleeping well. It is difficult to work. The first night after taking the new med, I went to bed at 10 p.m. and went right to sleep. Surprisingly, however, I woke up at midnight and was unable to go back to sleep. I watched TV but didn't get sleepy.

"Then I worked all day with only two hours' sleep. I felt awful and couldn't wait to get home. I was cranky and short with my co-workers. 'I know this has to get out today. I'm writing as fast as I can'!" I yelled at them.

"That night, I went to bed at ten and fell right to sleep—but woke up around midnight and couldn't get back to sleep. I felt terrible at work and short-tempered. This went on for two weeks as I waited for my follow-up appointment with you."

When she told him what was happening, Dr. Molina acknowledged, "That can't go on for long. Let's increase the dosage and try it another two weeks," he said.

The pattern remained the same. She said to herself, "I am not getting anything useful done when I sit up all night, so I might as well get something accomplished." Therefore, she started writing short stories at night.

At work, she was still bedraggled, whiny, and short-tempered while also inclined to make mistakes. Her new boss looked askance at her, but didn't say anything. Not able to tell anyone about her problem, knowing it was risking her job to say anything, she returned to Dr. Molina and told him, "That medication is still interrupting my sleep and it does not seem to be smoothing out my moods."

"Really? No help at all? That surprises me. I'll increase the dosage and see if that helps."

Marie knew it wouldn't help her so, desperate, she bought a bottle of wine. Marie was not a drinker and really didn't like to drink, but she needed sleep. Sure enough, by drinking several glasses of wine before bed she was able to sleep two more hours. However, it didn't seem to help her mood or acuity any. And it was worse at work.

Chapter Seventeen

When Marie went back to Dr. Molina's office, she told him about drinking wine to help her sleep.

"No, that doesn't help. Alcohol does not give you restful, rejuvenating sleep. It only complicates matters by making you more depressed. I had high hopes for this medication because the representative showed me such good results; but obviously, it is not right for you. However, it will take you three weeks to wean yourself off it. Then we can try something new. So keep taking it, but each week cut your dosage by 50 mgs. And stop drinking."

"Okay, but I just don't know how much longer I can take this," said Marie, running her hand through her hair.

"Don't worry, we'll figure it out. You know by now it is never easy to pinpoint a medication that will work for an individual."

Marie wasn't interested in putting on makeup or doing her hair nicely for work anymore. Her boss finally pulled her into her office and asked, "Why has your behavior changed so much? You are not doing your work as carefully, you look exhausted, and you aren't getting along with the others. Are you on drugs?"

Confronted so directly about her problems, Marie started to sob. "No, I have bipolar disorder and my meds stopped working. My doctor and I are trying to find a new medication and it takes time."

Ellen, an RN, didn't look startled or compassionate. She had a look of horror in her eyes and Marie knew immediately telling her was a mistake. Ellen was one of those who are afraid of mentally ill people; she didn't understand the disorder and was scared of what Marie would do.

Marie should have lied to her but the words were already out of her mouth. Within a week, she was stripped of her position as lead writer, and told that she would no longer manage the assignments or do extra work. Sometimes, if they were behind, Marie would come in on the weekends to get the work out on time. "Who will make the assignments?" she asked.

Ellen, said "I will, and everyone will do equal work."

"What if everything doesn't get done on time?"

"Then it won't get done." This was a complete turnaround from the attitude she had worked with for nine years. In the past, the goal was always to send a complete packet of work to the customer by the deadline.

"You will no longer prepare the syllabi for the printers. Flo will do that job and you will take over hers. Switch jobs with her immediately."

"But I am not sure exactly what she does…"

"You should know—you've been here long enough."

Marie went back to work, not feeling good about disclosure. She went to one of her former bosses, Bill, now a VP, and told him what happened. "Bill, I have bipolar disorder. I've had it since I started work here nine years ago. Recently my meds went bad on me and I am not doing well while I look for other medications. I believe that Ellen is going to fire me."

He said, "This doesn't sound right. I'll look into it for you."

Two days later Ellen called her in and told her, "You are not allowed to speak to Bill again. Stay completely away from him." She had the head of Personnel with her at the time.

The next week she was called back into Ellen's office. "You know, your proofing skills aren't up to par. You need to improve on them"

"That's been true for all the years I've worked here. I've leaned on the others for that and have written extra assignments to make up for it"

"That stops now. Everybody does the same work and you must be proficient in all of it."

Marie knew now she was being set up. Her anxiety level shot up, making it even more difficult to work mistake-free. Meanwhile Ellen hired Teresa so there would be more hands to manage the workload.

Dr. Molina started her on Paxil as an antidepressant, Topamax as a mood-stabilizer, and Risperdal to stop her mind from racing. The dosages were small at first, so she didn't feel any effect, and her behavior didn't change. She lived only a mile from work, so she asked, "Could I do some of my work at home? Maybe I wouldn't irritate people so much if I did, and I could be here in minutes if I were needed." This was met with a flat "No, that's impossible."

Marie soldiered on for several months, but nothing she did was right. In the spring, one day she was tormented by allergies and made drowsy by pills. She asked Ellen if she could go home sick; Ellen asked her to wait until after the staff meeting. Normally Ellen chaired the meeting, and then distributed an outline of it. This time was different—after the meeting, she asked Marie to make up the outline. Marie, who had been drowsing in the corner, was unable to do it.

Marie was being written up for her failings, and she had never before been written up in any job. She knew what was coming, but stayed in denial, not wanting to believe it. She had been fired from jobs before; but never one she loved as much as this one; one that was so much a part of her identity.

Cut out of the editing process, she did not always see mistakes, but once she caught Teresa's mistake that said exactly the opposite of what they meant to publish. Marie pointed it out to Ellen and all Ellen said was "okay." No praise or thanks.

She was incredulous the day Teresa told Ellen her husband's job was taking him to Florida so she would have to quit. To her astonishment, Ellen told Teresa they could arrange a way for her to work from Florida.

Marie was fired the next day.

Chapter Eighteen

It was sort of a relief finally to be fired, ending the uncertainty and the anxiety Marie had lived with for months. MedPrime gave her eighteen weeks of severance pay for the promise she wouldn't sue. Marie knew a suit would drag her through the mud and make her look bad; it would keep her upset for months or years. As a paralegal, she knew they would cite her illness as a reason for not doing quality work; they would point to her failings in proofing copy, point to her deterioration in grooming and ability to get along with others as signs of drug use. Therefore, she signed the papers and left. She felt awful about it all and lapsed into depression. Dr. Molina increased her antidepressant and that helped. In fact, it seemed that he had her on the right combination of drugs, because gradually she began to feel better.

"Listen," Dr. Molina's nurse told her the next time she went to the office, "Don't take this personally. We have another employee of your company going through the same thing you did. Sometimes it's just company policy."

"But I worked there nine years."

"It doesn't seem to count. They are always afraid a person with bipolar disorder will shoot up the place. Nothing you do will change their minds. It is just the stigma of mental illness."

Marie started looking for another job right away, hoping to get one before her severance pay ran out. However, after a while she began to believe that her age was working against her after going to job interview after job interview without success. Her appearance was impeccable and her demeanor cordial, but never got a job or second interview. She interviewed with periodicals, book producers, as a social worker, as a teacher. Not getting anywhere, and feeling so bad about losing Brad and her job, she stayed somewhat depressed for a year, even though she was on her meds.

Finally, she decided to get out of town, perhaps she could outrun her problems. She hired a moving company and relocated to Dallas, which was about four times bigger than Oklahoma City. She found an apartment in the north side of town. Oklahoma City was laid out in one day, the day of the Run, on a north-south grid pattern, and knowing the address of the place you wanted to go meant that you knew where it was. Dallas wasn't like that; it evolved over time and the street names didn't always follow a pattern or make sense. Buying a Mapsco, a detailed map of the city, and consulting it before she went anywhere, helped some.

She liked the vibrancy of the town and the life of the extensive downtown, but it was a bit overwhelming until she started to catch on to the rhythm of the town. She felt like a fish out of water for the first few months but was starting to find her way around town. She got her meds from the Mental Health Clinic because of not being able to afford a private doctor then.

Watching "Dateline" one night, she was floored to see a segment on the med Dr. Molina had put her on first. It seems the drug company had done testing on the med and discovered it had no effect on the treatment of bipolar disorder. Because they knew they could make a lot of money with a new bipolar medication, they marketed itas a new, effective bipolar med.

Marie was upset that a company would lie and take advantage of mentally ill people like that. She knew they wouldn't try that with a heart medication; there would be too much pushback from patients and the government. However, it wouldn't make that much difference if they took advantage of mentally ill people. No one would care.

No one ever cared what happened to the mentally ill. Marie Googled the drug and called the law firm who was doing the class action suit. She talked to a woman and told her about what the drug had done to her. The woman replied,

"I have heard your story over and over—people who took the medication and it had no effect so they had to ask for help at their job and were fired. That happened to dozens of people. Let me have you name and number and I'll let you know about the case."

~ * ~

A few weeks later, the woman from the law firm called back.

"We have so many people who were affected negatively by the drug we have decided to limit our clients to patients or families of patients who attempted or committed suicide while on the drug. I'm sorry, I know you suffered, too, but there are just too many people to handle all those who were damaged."

Marie called Dr. Molina and discussed it with him, and while he was circumspect in what he said about their experience with the drug, he maintained that he no longer considered it effective and that he had stopped prescribing it for patients about the same time she went off of it. Marie went off on a tirade about it, but he refused to say anything negative about the drug company. He just told her to be happy that they had found a combination that was working for her and to continue taking it. He wished her luck in her new life in Dallas.

Carleton

Chapter Nineteen

He strode down the street with his hands filled with dollar bills, holding them out to offer them to anyone within reach. Carleton David Chase was tall and loose-limbed, with brown hair, a pleasant, open face, and a big smile. There were no takers for the money as mothers clutched their children and backed away and men stared. Carleton had no clothes on.

After a few minutes, two policemen came up to him. They were a Mutt and Jeff team—one was fat and short, the other tall and skinny.

"Carleton, we thought that must be you when we got the call. C'mon now and get in the car. We'll go to the station and get you something to wear."

Carleton answered, speaking rapidly, "I wasn't doing anything. I was just trying to make people happy by giving them money."

"We know that, but sometimes people get the wrong idea when you don't wear any clothes. Now, please, come with us and we'll get you out of here."

"Well, okay."

Carleton crawled into the back seat of the squad car and chatted convivially. "How have you been since we last saw you?" asked the tall cop.

"Pretty good. I have a new band that I am playing with," answered Carleton.

"What's it like?"

"It's a Dixieland band. I saw their ad in the paper-- went and auditioned. They know I have bipolar disorder but said that didn't matter, only my piano playing mattered. They pick me up and drop me off for a gig because I don't have a car. One guy is a doctor, one a lawyer, and the other is a dentist."

"That sounds great," the tall cop said.

"Here we are. We're at the station. We are going to charge you with indecent exposure. After you are booked, the social worker will ask you for the name of your doctor and we'll get you straightened out."

"I don't want to go to jail."

"I know you don't, but it is the only way we can handle it. Maybe someday we'll have a better process."

As soon as they got in the jail, before they started the booking process, the cops got a white jumpsuit, marked on the back with "Dallas County Jail" to put on. It made Carleton feel like a criminal lawbreaker, but they were insistent he put it on before he was booked. Then he went through the whole booking process: fingerprinting, ID, charges recorded.

Carleton was placed in a cell by himself, even though he wanted to converse with other people. He asked the jailor nearest him, a young Hispanic man, holding his hands out beseechingly, "Why can't I go into the communal cell?"

"It's for your own good."

Carleton said, "Nothing will happen to me, I can take care of myself."

The jailor said, "They don't want to take chances with psychos like you."

"Who's a psycho? I am fine. Just watch me."

"Okay, I will."

Carleton didn't understand that at all and began to get angry, stating that he was arrested for no reason at all and now he was being held in solitary confinement. Almost immediately, the officers who brought him in came back to his cell and started talking with him.

"You know it scares people when you walk around with no clothing on and they always call us to come and get you. We've done this before. Once you are through court, they'll call your doctor, he'll give us a new dosage of your medication, and in a few days, you'll be able to go home. You just get out of whack every once in a while and need some help. You have done real well lately—it's been over a year since we've seen you. Please, just cooperate with us and we'll get you out of here as fast as possible."

Carleton calmed down with the familiar patrolmen and agreed he would cooperate. He found it impossible, though, to stand or sit still. He paced in his cell all through the day and night. He talked to any of the guards who would stop and speak with him, but he had lost a little of his bounce by the time it was time for him to go to court in the morning.

At court, the judge, who had thick black hair, a handlebar mustache and wore glasses, read out his charge of indecent exposure and before Carleton would plead, he asked him to define it for him. The judge asked him what he was doing when he was picked up, and Carleton told him, still speaking rapidly. "I took off my clothes and went out into the neighborhood to give people money. I wanted to help them out."

The judge said, "That is a perfect definition of it."

Carleton said, "I must be guilty, then, your honor."

"Five days," the judge said. "Have you talked with a social worker yet?

"No, I haven't."

The judge spoke to his staff in general, "Has he?"

The bailiff, a roly-poly little bald man in a uniform, answered, "No, I don't think so."

The judge turned to his clerk who was a middle-aged woman with dyed red hair, "Put him on the list. He needs his medicine."

The judge then moved on to the next person, and Carleton was taken back to his cell.

The other people in lockup were mostly winos with a few petty larcenies. Some of the men were still drunk, and most of them needed showers and new shoes. Carleton thought this isn't the right place for me; I should be in a hospital.

After a couple of hours, an obese young blond girl came to his cell. Standing outside the bars, she asked, "What's the name of your doctor and the mental health center where he works?"

"It's Dr. Russell at the Domain Mental Health Center," he snapped back. "But it would be easier to go through the psychiatric nurse."

"Does Dr. Russell have a phone number?"

Carleton strained to remember the number, wrinkled his brow, and inanely rubbed the side of his head as if it would help him to remember. The blond girl exhaled a sigh of impatience, crossed her arms, and scowled. Just as she started to turn away, Carleton exclaimed, "I got it — 863-5205."

"Thanks," said the girl, "I'll try to get your information this afternoon."

Carleton was not able to eat his supper and was now talking to himself, still pacing around his cell instead of sitting. He was making the jailors nervous, and they called the social worker to see what was happening. She told them she had a medication and a dosage and it would be dispensed that night.

When the nurse, a woman with stringy dyed black hair who looked like she was worn out, came, she gave Carleton some lithium, more than he had been taking. He had been without medication for two days, so it didn't slow him down, but the doctor told the nurse it would eventually. He continued to pace and chatter away to himself and to refuse food, but on the third day, he lay down in his bunk, drifted off to sleep, and slept for a full day. When he woke up, he seemed almost normal.

This was his last day to serve, so in the morning the jailors made sure he was fed his breakfast. "Carleton, we found these clothes and, while they aren't fancy, we think they will fit you well enough to get home in."

"Thanks, said Carleton, I was wondering about that."

He put on the clothes and checked his wallet. No one had taken any money from him, so he said,

"Good news, guys, I have enough money for train fare home."

As he left happily to go home, he said to all, in general, "Hope I don't see you again."

Chapter Twenty

As Carleton was growing up, he had a good relationship with his mother, a plump and kindly-faced woman with brown hair that was prematurely greying, but he could never seem to get along with his father. His father, who was skinny and tall, with black hair and eyes, wanted him to grow up and study business in college, but Carleton was only interested in music. It was the only thing he was interested in, and the only thing he wanted to do.

His mother paid for piano lessons, and Carleton was a genius on the piano. He took as much music as he could in the small schools he attended. He told his parents he wanted to go to music school instead of college, but his father wouldn't hear of it. He told Carleton, "You have to learn something that you can make a living at. Music is just a hobby, something you can have fun with, but you will never make a living with it. I will pay for business school but not for music."

The home he was raised in was modest, but sufficient. Carleton went without many of the things other children had, but he always had enough to eat and decent clothes to wear. They lived in a standard three bedroom, two-bath ranch style home that his mother had done her best to fix up with limited resources. Carleton knew his father was saving every extra penny so he could go to college.

Reluctantly, Carleton went to the small college his father chose for him, and enrolled in business courses. And he hated them. All his spare time was spent hooking up with other guys, forming bands and playing on the weekends. He didn't make much money, but he had a hell of a good time. Meanwhile, he was busy flunking out of his courses. At the end of the semester, he was told not to return to school. Carleton went home and told his dad, "I've flunked out of business school. Now will you let me go to music school?"

"No, absolutely not. I gave you your chance to get a good education and you blew it. Now you can leave my house and make your own way. I can't believe you are so ungrateful."

Carleton's mother cried as he packed and got ready to leave. They were in his bedroom; she gathered his things while he rejected them or placed them in his suitcases.

"Carleton, please write and tell me how you are getting on. I will be so worried about you if I don't hear from you. And, you know your father has his lodge meeting every Tuesday night; you could call me on those nights."

"I will, Mother, and I will study music."

"I hope you do. I know how good you are and how happy it makes you. I hope I see you soon, son."

Carleton put his arms around her and gave her a big hug. "I'm sorry, Mom, but you know I have to do this."

"Yes, son, I know you do."

Carleton headed straight for Massachusetts and the Berklee School of Music. He hopped a bus and made the long trip with others who were low on money and traveling light. He was superstitious about telling anyone where he was going; if anyone asked, he just said he was traveling up north to go to school.

When he got to Berklee, he went to the Counselor's Office and told the lady counselor:

"I have tried to study music all my life, but my father threw me out of the house when I failed business school. I have no money, but can you help me find work or something so I can go to school here?"

The counselor asked him a few more questions, and when she learned how he had studied music all his life and been rejected by his father for it, she said, "We'll let you audition for three of the professors, and see how you do. We can make a decision after that."

The day of the audition, Carleton was scared. It was held in the auditorium, with only Carleton and three of the music professors present. Carleton's steps echoed on the stage when he walked out to meet them. They introduced themselves solemnly, without even a smile of encouragement. Carleton was so afraid his hands shook. He took a deep breath, and then started to play. The professors listened to him play the piano, mostly contemporary music, and finally pronounced him extraordinarily talented and worth their efforts. They went to work and got him a full scholarship to the school, which was one of the premier contemporary music schools in the country.

When they called Carleton in and told him the news, he could hardly speak. He sputtered to the professors and the Dean of the School. "Ohmigod! I have, I have wanted to go to Berklee as long as my life. As long as I can remember. This is a dream come true for me. Thank you, thank you so much for this opportunity. I won't let you down, I promise."

Carleton got himself a string of minimum wage jobs as he went to school, and while he had the opportunity, soaked up all he could learn about music. Still he was best on the piano, and he dazzled everyone with his talent and added to his ability by learning everything he could. He was an excellent student who made his teachers enjoy teaching him all that they could. When he graduated, the Dean said,

"We are so proud of how well you have done. You certainly made the scholarship worth it."

Carleton made it a point to thank the Dean and all of his teachers for giving him the chance to learn. After graduation, he headed to Los Angeles, since he had always wanted to work for Walt Disney. He thought they did the best and most varied work in music; he also thought it would be a good place to get a job. He went to Walt Disney Studios in Burbank, where he gave them his résumé and demonstrated his ability.

He got through the interview and had an audition set up. Afterward at the successful audition, he stunned the music director and the producers. "Wow, we can really use you. When can you start?" the music director said.

Carleton agreed to start right away and called his mother that Tuesday night to give her the good news. He called her from a bar in the neighborhood where he had settled. He was nervous, not knowing how the job was going to work out, but she was proud of him for making his way through school, and now was over the moon about his new job. Carleton said, "Now don't tell Dad about the job."

"Why, Carleton, this will just show him that you were right and he was wrong?"

"I don't know, something just tells me not to brag about it yet. But I know I will do a good job and that it will be really fun."

"Keep calling me, Carleton, and let me know how things go. I am so proud of you!"

Carleton was so happy to get a job with a company like Disney. There were always projects going on, and he worked on several. He was on a salary and was on call whenever they needed him. He was also allowed to give input on his job when it was needed.

After he had been working for about six months and had garnered a reputation as a reliable, talented musician, Carleton began to feel funny. Everything seemed to slow down around him. His producer told him, "Carleton you are playing too fast. You are throwing off the other players and generally making a mess of this scene."

"Okay," said Carleton, "I'll slow down."

But he didn't. He kept playing as fast as before and then even faster. The producer, Evan, who was young, impatient, and openly gay, lost his cool and sent everyone home.

The next day was even worse. Carleton hadn't been able to get any sleep and was really revved up. His playing was way too fast and he was ruining the show. Evan said,

"Carleton, you are not in sync with the rest of the group and the music. Now get with the program!"

"I'm trying Evan, I'm trying. I'll get it this time."

But Carleton couldn't seem to comply.

Raising his voice, Evan almost shouted, "Just get out of here, you're fired!"

Chapter Twenty-One

Carleton was confused and couldn't seem to straighten out his thinking. Evan told him he was playing too rapidly and messing up the whole program, but Carleton thought he was playing normally. He felt so bad about losing his first real job that he couldn't eat or sleep. At night, he couldn't contain himself, so he walked the streets, with stops at greasy little diners for coffee.

His thoughts were racing and he couldn't slow them down. After several days with no food or sleep, he decided that he wanted to help his neighbors out, even though he was miserable, so he took off his clothes, walked outside with handfuls of dollar bills, and tried to give them away. Everyone cringed away from him and after a few minutes, a cop car drove up next to him, the patrolmen got out and one of them asked, "What do you think you are doing?"

Carleton answered, his words coming fast, "I'm just helping out the world, giving money to people who might need it."

"You better come with us; we've had some complaints about you."

"What kind of complaints?"

"That you are out here on the street doing things you shouldn't."

There was a crowd of people staring at him by now, and the cops were insistent. So Carleton got into the car and the police took him to a hospital, a big one. He was checked in and given a tiny room. When he still wouldn't eat or sleep, a young, foreign doctor examined him and, after about five minutes, told him and the nurse with him that he had bipolar disorder.

"You are extremely manic and unable to function. However, a regimen of lithium should straighten you out in a number of days. Nurse, let's start him on 800 milligrams until he smooths out. Carleton, you'll be fine."

Carleton didn't know what bipolar disorder was, but he was thinking too rapidly to care. He paced all day and the nurses let him walk the halls all night. He was given a sedative the first night, but it didn't seem to help. During the day, he couldn't concentrate enough to participate in group therapy or games or even to sit and watch TV. The nurses talked with him when they had time and listened to his ramblings, but didn't try to reason with him.

Carleton told them, "I am a musician and I played for Walt Disney. I used to make a lot of money doing projects and movies for him, but he didn't like me or my piano playing, I don't know why. I tried hard to please Evan but for some reason I couldn't make him happy. I tried and I tried. When I get out of here, I will go back to work there, but not for Evan, no, not for him. I'll work for a different producer, one who understands me, and everything will work out again. I can't believe Evan fired me for no reason. I was trying to play the way he wanted me to. I tried as hard as I could."

The nurses would sympathize with him and go on about their work. After about the fourth or fifth day, Carleton started to slow down and to realize that he had been ill. At that time, Dr. Patel had a talk with him and explained, "You have bipolar disorder. It is a cyclical disease and cycles differently for each person. You will have to take lithium for the rest of your life to control the illness; with it, you should be fine. The course of the illness is different for everyone, but for someone like you, lithium should keep you stable."

"I don't understand why I lost my job."

"You became manic, or speeded up. Your thoughts began racing, and your actions followed. You were doing everything fast—talking, playing. Finally, you went into a psychotic state in which you thought you could help people by giving them your money."

"Can I get my job back?"

"You can try, but I doubt it. Once you have acted out like that, people are afraid of you. I would suggest that you find another town to work in where no one knows about your reputation. I'm sorry, but the stigma against the illness is so strong that it is best that you control it with no one knowing you have it. We will let you out of the hospital in a couple of days and you can go on from there."

While Carleton was in the hospital, he wrote his mother and told her the whole story so she wouldn't worry any more, since she hadn't heard from him in a while. He knew it would be a blow to her but thought it would be best that she know the truth. The doctor told him it was hereditary; maybe it explained some of his father's strangeness. After he got out of the hospital, with a supply of lithium and an appointment with the Mental Health Center, he was sad and depressed about losing his job. He knew he had talent. It was upsetting that an illness would derail his career like this.

He cried about his situation, and then decided he better act on the doctor's advice. He sold everything and got up some cash, then had to figure out where to move. He knew Austin, Texas, was a place with lots of live music, so he set his sights there. Carleton was nervous and afraid of what the future held for him, but he started for Austin with his hopes high now that he knew what his problem was and how to control it. It was a two-day drive and he was tired when he got there, but he sought out the clubs on Sixth Street and talked with band members. After a few days, he had some leads. When he followed up on these, he was hired on with the "Platinum Fans."

The lead singer, Ashley, who had shoulder-length blond hair, asked him where he worked before, and he said, "Walt Disney."

"What happened there?"

"Well, they were just too straight for me. Too much structure. You know how it is."

"Cool," said Ashley. "Welcome aboard."

Things were looking up. He meshed well with the band members, both socially and music-wise. Carleton could play any kind of contemporary music, so he fit in well. They didn't have gigs every night, but played almost every weekend. They had a few albums out, and one of them was selling well. Carleton took a small apartment and soon learned his way around town. He gained a reputation as a stand-up guy who stayed away from drugs.

For eight months, Carleton and the band did well. Then, all of a sudden, Ashley was telling him that he was playing too fast and messing up the music. A shudder went through Carleton. He didn't perceive his playing to be any faster than before. He did, however, deliberately try to slow down his playing; but the other band members continued their complaints. They also said he was talking too loud and fast, and that he wasn't listening to them when they made plans for gigs.

Carleton made an emergency appointment at the Mental Health Center of Travis County. Dr. Ahmed talked for him for a few minutes, then had a social worker drive him over to the hospital after he told him, "Carleton, you are way manic. I mean, off-the-chart. You have to go to the hospital to get straightened out."

"But I've been taking my lithium."

"Evidentially your mania broke through the lithium. At the hospital, they will care for you and step up your dosage.

The dosage will be too high for you to handle by yourself—but, you'll be okay."

Carleton went to the hospital and, again, couldn't eat or sleep. He was slowly brought down through the administration of high doses of lithium, and then released. He went straight to his apartment, where he was told he had been evicted because of non-payment of rent.

He then looked up the band. Ashley told him that because of his weird behavior and his disappearance, they had replaced him. They didn't trust him enough to want him back. Carleton thought he was pretty much done in Austin, so he packed up what little he had and moved to Dallas.

Chapter Twenty-Two

When Carleton got home after his stay in jail in Dallas, the guys in his rooming house were happy to see him. They were also happy to see the mind-blowing fast-talking, fast acting, no-sleeping, no-eating behavior had gone. The first thing Carleton wanted to do was to see his kitten. He started for his room, saying, "I can't wait to see Blackie."

He heard feet shuffling and then,

"Carleton, we didn't know when or if you were going to come back," said Bruce, "so we took your kitten to the pound. I'm sorry."

"You did what? Couldn't you have kept her for me? Blackie didn't eat much. Now it is too late to get her back. She has either been killed or adopted by now."

"We just didn't know what to do. We did what we thought best for the kitten."

Carleton turned his back and stomped to his room. Inside, the only things left of Blackie were her empty food and water bowls, her dirty litter box, and some toys scattered around. He was angry; seems that with all else, he couldn't even own a cat, couldn't take care of one. He would never get one again.

Carleton knew he had ruined himself in this neighborhood, so he packed up and moved to the McKinney Avenue area, where there were a lot of expensive clubs and cheaper apartments in the Knox-Henderson neighborhood. He was also a short bus ride from Deep Ellum, which was another club area, catering to the younger crowd.

Carleton was able to pick up gigs in both areas, playing several instruments, but the piano stayed his first love. He asked, "Will you pay me under the table?" He wanted this, so it didn't mess up his Supplemental Social Security Income, which was a small government grant he applied for and received right after he moved to Dallas.

He started going to the Mental Health Center in Dallas as soon as he got there. The personnel there helped him with the paperwork, and he was assigned to Dr. Bodapapi, who looked the part of an Indian psychiatrist. After listening to Carleton's story, he said, "If you can recognize the symptoms of mania coming, you can come to the clinic and get an additional dosage of your lithium. Lithium controls you for months at a time so I really believe that it is the best medication for you."

"That would help a lot, but I never realize that I am manic until I have already acted out. I wish I could recognize the early stages. I can't hold a job for any length of time and I really do want to work."

"I suggest you keep a journal in which you record your actions and feelings every day. That might tip you off to something unusual coming up."

"Thanks for the idea, Dr. Bodapapi, I will try that. That could make the difference. Right now the SSI allows me to live, but I would like to play again in a regular band."

"Give it try and let me know."

Carleton tried keeping a journal, but found that when he started getting manic, he stopped journaling. Finally, one night in Deep Ellum, he took off all his clothes. Luckily, it was such an avant-garde neighborhood that it didn't ruin his reputation or keep him from further jobs. They just thought he was a little wacky. It frustrated him, though, because he couldn't find a solution.

The next time he went to the doctor, he again asked for a solution. "Is there any way I can prevent going manic? Nothing I've tried so far has worked."

"I'm going to set your appointments only a month apart, so maybe we can help you catch the mania. I'm also going to start you on supplemental medications to try to keep you stable. I want you to work as badly as you do. Get your meds downstairs and keep trying. Good luck," said Dr. Bodapapi.

Carleton did get on with a band, a Dixieland band formed by professionals, a doctor, a dentist, and a lawyer, who played part-time. It wasn't much, but it gave him an identity and a band that he could say he worked for. It didn't pay a lot, but it was home. It improved his mood, and having appointments once a month with the Center meant that twice in a year his mania was caught early. Things were looking up for him and he hoped it continued.

Conversations

Chapter Twenty-Three

It was less expensive to go to the Mental Health Clinic than to a private doctor, but it could take longer to be seen and to get meds. Often patients would fall into conversation with each other, comparing doctors, medications, symptoms, and stories. Four regulars on Tuesday evenings struck up a friendship, and asked one other,

"Wouldn't it be fun to meet during the week just to talk things over?" said Marie.

"Oh, yeah," said Suzy, "just about the time we get into a good conversation one of us has to go in for her appointment."

"Well, I know I would like to talk to you guys more," said Abby.

"I know," said Missy, "let's meet at one on Wednesdays for coffee at the Denny's on Lemmon and Inwood. That way we'll have enough time to talk. We can be a 'support group' without the clinic ever knowing!"

Before anyone could answer, a tall guy two rows in front of them leaned back and said,

"Can I join?"

"Well, so far it's just women, but if you don't mind that, sure, you can come." Suzy spoke up and said, "I have a friend you will all like. Can we include her, too?"

Marie chimed in, "I don't see why not."

The next day Marie, Carleton, Missy, and Abby commandeered the large booth in back. The restaurant looked like every Denny's in the country, clean and casual with friendly servers. A few minutes later Suzy came in with a tall blond whom she introduced as "Jackie." They greeted her and made introductions all around. Carleton explained that he had to take the bus, but it wasn't that far. "Yeah, Carleton, I have to take the bus, too, and it is a long trip for me. My car was repossessed," Missy said.

"Oh, no," the group chorused.

It was summer in Dallas, and the heat was oppressive—the temperature in the 100s. Everyone ordered a Diet Coke. Marie laughed and said, "I never knew anyone with bipolar disorder who wasn't addicted to Diet Coke. If Coke knew how much we supported them, maybe they would make a donation."

"I know, I drink it all day long in the summer; maybe I'll have coffee in the morning in the winter, but Diet Coke the rest of the day," said Missy

"I buy it in those big 3-liter bottles and drink half of one a day," countered Marie.

"Well, whatever we do, we don't mess around with it, we go all out," said Carleton.

Abby asked, "Do you think we should have any rules?"

Missy spoke up, "No, we aren't really a support group. We're just here because we are friends and want to talk to each other."

Abby said, "I have questions for some of you who have been on medication longer. I have just been diagnosed and don't know too much about it."

"That's fine. No problem. Of course we can talk about being bipolar; that's what we have in common," Marie said.

"Sure," "Okay," "Right," said the others.

"Let me start off," said Abby.

"I am just back from a year in France. While I was there, I was attending veterinary school and I fell in love with a married man. We broke up when he wouldn't leave his family, but I am so obsessed with him that I want to go back to France even though I know that would be foolish. I just can't get over him."

"I know how you feel," Marie said. "I have been there. I dated a guy for ten years who cheated on me and when he finally committed to me, he scared himself and dumped me without a word. I stayed obsessed with him for years until I got on the right medications. So trust me, all you have to do is find your medications, and that entire obsession will go away."

"Really?" said Abby. "That sounds wonderful."

"Just don't give up. Keep trying until you get the meds. If you give up, you'll never get anywhere. I know it is frustrating, but just keep trying."

"Is it really that easy?" asked Missy.

"No, I didn't mean to make it sound easy. It can take five weeks or five years to find the right medication. There is no test that tells you what medication to take. You have to get on a med, see if it works by staying on it a few weeks, and if it doesn't, it takes about three weeks to get off it. Some people just can't take all this and they flat give up. You can't do that because you'll never get there if you do. But it is so frustrating. It is much easier now than it was when I did it twenty years ago," said Marie.

The waitress interrupted, "You folks want to order?"

"Thanks, Marie. That really makes me feel better."

Jackie said, "I think I'll have a salad."

"Me, too," said Suzy.

"Not me," said Carleton, "I'm having a burger."

Suzy spoke up, "I have been trying to get the right dosage of meds for a couple of years, but I haven't succeeded yet. I was in love with a rock star and he loved me, but he died and I miss him so. He loved me so much— he died with my picture in his hand."

"Who was he?" Abby asked.

"Emmanuel Sanchez. He was on the David Letterman show a lot."

"I don't watch those late-night shows, sorry," said Marie.

"You all would have liked him if you had seen him," said Suzy.

Carleton and Jackie had heard of him, but none of the others had. Suzy said, "Would you like it if I made CDs of his music for you?"

"Oh I already have one, and it is great," said Jackie.

Carleton said, "I would like that."

"I would love that," said Missy.

Marie said, "That would be very nice of you."

"I would want one, too," said Abby.

How long ago did he die?" asked Marie.

"It's been two years. I still miss him constantly."

"It sounds like you might be obsessed with him," Marie observed.

"No, I'm not. I just love him."

"I don't know, Suzy, that could be obsession," said Marie.

"I tell you, I am not obsessed with him. I just loved him and miss him a lot."

"Jackie, you haven't said a word. Tell us about you," said Abby.

"It's kind of a long story. I was involuntarily committed by the cops, and when I was in the hospital I was raped."

"No—who raped you?" Missy exclaimed. Carleton's fork clattered on the floor. Missy and Abby gasped.

"Another patient?" asked Marie

"No, I think it was a staff member, but I am not sure. No one at the hospital believed me, and I couldn't really deal with it then because I was trying to get out. I've had some therapy since then but I am still terrified of going to the hospital. Afterwards I just lay on the couch and watched TV for a year."

"I guess so, that's awful, "said Abby.

"Why were you committed?" asked Marie.

"I drove the wrong way down a one-way street and had an accident. Totaled my brand-new car."

"Why would you do that?" asked Abby.

"I just wanted to. It seemed like a good idea at the time."

"Ah, the anthem of the bipolar—It Seemed Like a Good Idea at the Time," said Carleton.

"Oh, yeah," said Marie.

Missy said, "I am so sorry,"

Suzy said, "It gets worse, you all."

"Oh, no, said Marie"

Carleton was silent, but alert.

Jackie said, "I've made my peace with that because I have no other choice, but that isn't the worst thing that happened to me at the hospital. I gave my parents temporary custody of my son and they took me to court and made it permanent custody by convincing the judge that I am an unfit mother. And one of the things they used against me was that I imagined I was raped!"

"Jackie, that is terrible. How could they do that to you?" said Missy.

"They think they are helping my son, David, but I believe they are using him to replace the son they lost. My brother committed suicide and they are showering David with things, things that I couldn't afford to give him. They have convinced the court that I am not capable of caring for him because I am crazy. It makes me so sad."

"I would think it would make you mad," said Missy.

"That, too," said Jackie.

"I guess you can't afford to go to court and convince them that you are capable of caring for him," Abby said.

"No, I can't, and I have to stay on good terms with them so I can have access to David. They do help me with money, too—but it is the least they can do."

"I'm sorry, Jackie," said Missy.

Jackie had started to tear up, so Marie turned the attention to Carleton. "Carleton, you haven't said anything. What do you do?"

"I'm on SSI, but I also work part time in a band."

"Cool, what kind of band?" asked Marie

"It's a Dixieland band and the other members are professionals who just do it for fun. We get a few gigs and I make a little money."

"That sounds like fun," said Abby.

"It is, but I would like to play fulltime."

"Why don't you?"

"I get too manic to keep a fulltime job."

"I know that feeling," said Missy.

Missy, you haven't told us anything about yourself. What is your story?" asked Suzy.

"I don't think I am ready to yet. Maybe next week."

"On that note, I have to leave. Time to wash my hair," stated Jackie.

"I have to get home and cook dinner for my mother— she'll be home from work soon," said Missy.

"Okay, same time next week?" said Marie.

There was a chorus of "yeses" and "okays."

"Wait," said Jackie. "Let's exchange e-mails and phone numbers so we can get in touch if we need to,"

That seemed like a good idea, so with a little confusion, everyone except Jackie and Suzy, who already knew the others' information, exchanged their e-mail addresses and phone numbers.

They all stepped into the heat and went their separate ways.

Chapter Twenty-Four

It was hot again the next Wednesday they met. They ordered Diet Coke, and put in food orders. Then the talk started---

"Listen, I have a problem and need advice. I have to go to court on a DWI next month. What am I going to do? I don't want to interrupt my treatment by going to jail—and I don't want to go to jail at all. What can I do?" a nervous, shaking Missy asked.

"I know," said Jackie, "get your doctor to write a letter to the court stating that you have bipolar disorder and are getting treatment for it. Have him say how you never miss an appointment and how hard you are working to get well. That should help a lot. There are few advantages to having bipolar disorder, but every once in a while it at least helps us to explain our situation, if the person is willing to listen."

"Be sure to tell him to say that you are cooperative and improving," said Suzy.

"I am cooperative—I am trying my best---but I don't think I am improving at all."

"What are you taking?" asked Marie.

"Effexor and something else, I don't know."

"If you have been on them for six weeks and they are not helping, ask your doctor to try something else. Describe your symptoms to him exactly," said Jackie.

"How did you get a DWI?" asked Suzy.

"I was drinking a fifth of vodka a day, so how did I get only one? I had a good job, a nice car, and an apartment, but I lost everything. I was so manic, and I was really in love with this guy. Turned out he had two baby mamas. I thought he really cared about me, but I was just another woman to him. The whole thing was really awful."

"How did you lose everything? It sounds terrible," asked Marie.

"I was evicted three times, my car was repossessed, and I just stopped going to work. I was drunk all the time and didn't care about anything. The only things I hung onto were my cell phone and my cat."

"God, Missy, I hope you get on the right meds soon. It sounds like you really need them. I don't know anyone else who has been that manic," said Marie.

"Except for me," interjected Carleton. Abby, Marie, Suzy, and Jackie brushed his comment off.

"How long did it take you, Marie, to get properly medicated?" asked Missy.

"It took five years from the time I was diagnosed until I got on the right meds. They kept me on lithium and kept telling me that it was working, even though I kept telling them that it wasn't. They said I just didn't know that it was working; is that crazy or what? I had to go to a hospital, to their Affective Disorders Unit, to get proper treatment. That med lasted me for twelve years, until my husband died and I got fired."

"Is everyone on disability?" Missy asked the group.

"No, I'm not," said Abby.

"But I am," said Carleton,

"Me, too, said Suzy

Jackie said, "I am, too."

"How do you get it?" said Missy.

"You just go to the Social Security website and apply. It is a long, drawn-out application, but I never saw anyone who needed it more than you do," said Jackie.

"I almost forgot, "said Suzy, "I have your CDs of Manny's songs in my tote bag. I burned one for each of you."

Each took one and said, "Thanks."

"I hope you enjoy them," said Suzy, "I think he is really good. Did I tell you he died with my picture in his hand?"

"Yes, you did," said Marie. "What did he die of?"

"Lung cancer."

"Oh, no, that makes me want to quit smoking."

"Missy, you should stop smoking. It took me twenty-five years, and smoking that long did me no good," said Marie.

"Yes, Missy, you should stop. I smoked for a long time and now I have emphysema. It will eventually kill me," said Carleton.

Missy raised her voice. "For God's sake, I just quit drinking and lost my lover, and you want me to give up smoking, too. I am so worried about that damn DWI and about having no income and having to live with my mom. There is no way I could quit smoking right now. I can't believe you are on my back about it. I don't need this. Just lay off!"

"Missy, I am so sorry," said Marie. "I quit smoking years after I got on my medications. There is no way in hell that someone who is still trying to get medicated can quit." Missy picked out a tress of her hair and started to twist it around one of her fingers. "One of the hardest things a person with bipolar can do is to quit smoking. It was rude of me and Carleton to even mention it to you. It is something you can take care of when you are ready. Yes, you should stop smoking, but you should not even think about it now. I am sorry."

Missy still looked offended. She shook her head and said, "You know how hard it is. You smoked while you were unmedicated. I can't believe you preach to me about something you couldn't have done," Missy sniffed. She was so angry that tears had come to her eyes. Carleton apologized, too, and Missy calmed down.

"Most people with bipolar disorder smoke, and you can't quit until you are stable, so don't worry about it now," said Marie.

"I want to tell you, doctors put me on lithium and told me it was working. Then they put me on anti-psychotics on top of the lithium. I was taking an antidepressant on top of all that. I was a real mess. Nothing quite like too many of the wrong drugs. Now they are much better about trying you on different medications, and they have so many to choose from. I wish they had a blood test to tell you what meds to take, but it is all trial and error."

Carleton broke in, "I have been on lithium for years, and it works great for me. In fact, it's the only thing that works for me. I'm lucky, 'cause it's really cheap."

"You must be more of the 'classic' type of bipolar, Carleton. For the longest time physicians thought only lithium would work. It's only been a few years ago since they realized anti-seizure meds, like I take, will work for those who lithium doesn't help."

"My meds are really working well for me," said Jackie. "I think I am going back to school in the fall, if I can get that rape out of my head and convince my parents to give me weekends with David."

Jackie, that would be great!" said Suzy. "Do you think you can do it?"

"I'm working with the therapist on getting past the rape, and my parents seem to be letting up on me. I think if they see me going back to school they might think I can handle things more responsibly."

"Where would you go to school and what would you major in?' asked Abby.

"I'm just thinking about starting at Richland Junior College, and I haven't decided on a major yet. I feel so much calmer and ready to take on new things. I have wasted the past two years; now at least I am out of my parents' home and on my own. If only I had David with me!"

"Gee, I'm living with my mother now and it does drive a person crazy, but at least I had somewhere to go," said Missy.

"There is that," agreed Jackie.

"I would have lived on the street rather than go home to my parents, but I could have lived with my mother," said Marie. "My father was impossible. I stayed until I was 18, and then got out for good."

"Mine weren't that bad, said Suzy. They got me a house and paid for it. When I was so much sicker and thought there were cameras in my home, spying on me, they put up with me. I know it wasn't easy for them. I was so paranoid."

"Now, I have never thought anything like that," said Marie.

"She was in bad shape," said Jackie. "She even smashed the smoke alarms because she thought they were cameras."

"You must have been scared," said Missy.

"Yes, I was, but I have improved a great deal and am still getting better."

"I guess it's time to go, but Missy, you hang in there," said Marie.

"Okay, but it is really hard. I sometimes think it is better to be manic."

"No, Missy, don't start thinking like that. Remember the havoc you wreaked last time.

"Oh, I do, and I won't go through that again."

"All of us are pulling for you, Missy; I know you will make it," said Jackie, "and we'll check on you next week."

Chapter Twenty-Five

When the group got together next, Abby, said with a big smile, "I have an announcement to make."

"What is it?" "Tell us." "Did you meet someone?" chorused the group.

"No, it is good news, though. My meds kicked in two days ago. That awful anxiety went away and I am no longer obsessing about the guy in France. In fact, I don't think about him anymore. I have no desire to go back to France and see him now. You have no idea what freedom that is. I was so anxious and so torn-up about him I just couldn't stay with my parents. They were trying so hard to make me feel better it was driving me nuts so I came out here to stay with my ex-roommate. She encouraged me to go to the Mental Health Center and you guys encouraged me to stay with it. I am going back to school at Virginia Tech and I want to spend a little time with them before I do. My flight to Connecticut leaves tomorrow morning."

"Abby, that is great," said Marie, "I am glad you got straightened out so fast. I told you it would work."

"I am so happy for you. I wish my meds were working that fast," said Missy.

"Congratulations!" said Jackie. "Now you know what it's like to be stable."

"I'm right behind you," said Suzy.

"It is a good feeling, isn't it," said Carleton.

"Well, I can't stay any longer today. I just didn't want to leave without telling you and thanking all of you. I have your e-mail addresses so we can stay in touch. I am so excited to be going back to school. For a while, I didn't think I could make it. And this year I spend most of my year on my specialty, horses. I just can't wait."

Abby stood up to leave and they all wished her "good luck" and a "safe trip." Afterwards, Marie said, "I will really miss Abby," and everyone agreed with her. It was heartening to see someone respond well to medication and to be so happy.

Jackie remarked, "Missy, you don't look happy. I know your meds aren't working yet, but they will, you just have to keep plugging away."

"That's part of it, but my doctor changed my meds this week and I can't afford to buy them. I don't see how I will ever get better this way," Missy said.

"What did he put you on?" asked Suzy

"Topamax."

"That's no problem," said Marie. "When I first moved to town and started going to the clinic, they must have had a surplus of Topamax. They gave me this sack full of bottles of it. Since then I've been getting prescriptions for it from a doctor who didn't know I had such a stash. In fact, I told her I did, but she really doesn't believe I have this much and she keeps giving me more. So, this afternoon I'll give you a ride home. We'll stop by my apartment and pick up some pills for you."

"That would be great," said Missy.

"Keep in mind, this is completely illegal, and we could get in a lot of trouble for doing this, so let's just keep it among the group. But to me it sounds like a good solution to your problem," said Marie.

Just then, someone in the kitchen dropped a whole tray of dishes, and everyone jumped. The noise was awful. "Gosh, I wonder if they have already caught on to us," said Marie.

"It would help me out a lot," said Missy.

"Sounds good to me," said Jackie. I wouldn't say a word because I might need help like that sometime."

"Me, too." said Suzy.

"Hey, I'm not proud," agreed Carleton.

"But tell me about how it works," said Missy.

"The good news," Marie said, "is that it causes you to lose rather than gain weight, so it offsets those meds that put weight on."

"Great," said Missy, "and the bad news…"

"The bad news is that it causes word-finding problems."

"What does that mean?" asked Missy.

"You'll be talking along, and all of a sudden you won't be able to remember a common word. You'll know it; you just won't be able to say it. It's really weird," said Marie.

"Sounds like it," said Missy.

"It is a really funny feeling and after a few minutes you can usually come up with the word. Meanwhile, people are finishing your sentences for you," said Marie, "but it works really well for me and the fact that it doesn't add to your weight is a real plus."

"Did you get your application in for Social Security Disability?" asked Suzy.

"Yes, and what a pain. How long does it take to get it?" asked Missy.

"We can't answer that question. It all depends," said Marie.

"I got mine right away," said Carleton, "but of course it is SSI because I hadn't worked enough quarters to get Social Security Disability."

"It took me about four months, not really long at all. But it seems like forever when you don't have any money coming in," Jackie said.

"It didn't take me long at all," said Suzy. "You can hope that it will be fast for you, too.'

"Hey, I forgot to ask how you liked the CDs I made for you all. What did you think?" interjected Suzy.

"I really liked the songs, thanks, Suzy," said Jackie

"My favorite one was 'For My Second Trick," said Marie.

Carleton said, "I liked them all."

"I really appreciated your making it for me, Suzy," said Missy.

"I'm glad you liked them," said Suzy, "I think they are wonderful."

"Carleton, you probably appreciated them more than anyone else, being a musician and all," said Marie.

"Yes, I really liked them."

"Well, I have to be going," said Jackie, "great seeing all of you."

"Come on, Missy, I'll take you home, "said Marie.

"Sure beats the bus," answered Missy.

They went out to the parking lot and waved "good-bye" to the others. The car was stiflingly hot but that's why they made air conditioning. Everyone in Texas, just about, had it in their home and car. As soon as it cooled down a little and Marie got away from the busy corner, she asked Missy, "Do you really think Suzy had such a big love affair with Manny as she says?"

"No, I really don't. I think it was just a passing thing. But you know what? There is a biography of him coming out next month and I read a review that said it is all about the many women in his life."

"Interesting—I'll have to get a copy of that."

"What did you really think of the CD, Marie?

"I kind of like it, but it is not really my style—I'm into oldies and more mainstream pop, but there is no reason to tell Suzy that. She loves everything about him"

"I felt the same way," said Missy.

By that time, they had reached Marie's apartment. They went in, and Marie said, "Do you want a Coke?"

"No, I think I finally had enough at Denny's."

"Okay, just let me find those pills."

Missy looked around the apartment. It was small, one-bedroom, with a contemporary couch covered with an abstract design in muted colors and a handsome mahogany desk that held her computer. She saved the furniture from her marriage. Missy picked up the picture of a young man on the desk next to the computer and asked, "Is this a picture of your son on the desk?"

Marie called back from the bathroom, "No, that's my stepson, Ben." She came back into the living room. "Here, I have packaged these pills in a box and I'll stuff the box with newspaper to keep them from rattling. Now they sound just like pills. Just in case we get stopped," she said with exaggerated drama. She rattled the box to demonstrate.

She took the "Dallas Morning News" and balled up pages of it, stuffing them into the box. Soon she could shake the box all she wanted and it was soundless. "Okay, let's get you home. I know you have to start supper for your mom, and I don't want to get caught in traffic on the way back."

Chapter Twenty-Six

The Denny's where they met was quieter than usual when they got together the next Wednesday. Right away, Suzy said, "Jackie called me. She won't be able to make it today. She had something to do with David."

"Okay," said Missy.

"All right," said Marie.

"I hope she's okay," said Carleton.

"She is," said Suzy, "she'll be back next week."

"I've had a problem, said Marie. I have two cats, Charlie and Camilla. It's been hard enough for them to adjust to apartment living, but we got a new manager last week and she just decided that cats could no longer go outside. Camilla is down with it, but Charlie is having a hard time. All this time he has always gone out whenever he wanted and now he has to stay in."

"That's just impossible," said Missy. "My Strad is an inside cat, but I can't imagine convincing an outside cat to stay in."

"Well, Charlie is pretty smart. He knows lots of English words. He even knows what I mean when I say, 'Just a minute.' I've been letting him go out early in the morning and late in the evening and he is already catching on, though it is hard for him."

"I love cats. I wish I could have one," said Carleton.

"Why can't you?" asked Missy.

"What happens if I get manic and have to go to the hospital and have to leave it?"

"Won't your neighbors take care of it while you're gone?" asked Marie.

"No, I've already been through that. I had a little black kitten and when I went to jail, they took it to the pound. I just can't have a kitten."

"I'm sorry, Carleton, that is really awful."

"I'm sorry, too," said Missy.

"You know, I really miss Manny. I loved him so much, and it was just so hard when he died," said Suzy.

"I'm sure it was hard for you, Suzy. It is always hard to lose someone you love. I had a man leave me without a word after ten years and I was bent out of shape for years over that," said Marie.

"But he loved me so much; he died with my picture in his hand. I just miss him a lot," said Suzy.

"I know you do, Suzy, I'm sorry you have to go through this," said Missy.

"Sometimes his songs get stuck in my head and I hear them all the time," said Suzy.

"Oh, that is awful. That happened to me one time when I was really manic and it drove me crazy," said Marie.

"I like it. I like being able to hear his voice all the time. It is comforting to me," said Suzy.

Missy and Marie exchanged a glance. Then Marie spoke up. "You know, I live alone and really don't want to cook. Does anyone have an idea for lunch that isn't a sandwich and is easy to fix?"

Suzy looked hurt, but didn't say anything about the sudden change of subject. She just said, "I'm into vanilla yogurt with pecans right now."

"Hey, that sounds good," said Marie.

"Yeah, you'll have us all eating that," said Missy.

"Jackie started last week," said Suzy.

"Oh, I wanted to tell you," Missy said. "I can't really tell that the Topamax is helping yet, but I was trying to say something to my mother last night about the air conditioner and I could NOT think of the word for 'thermostat.' I kept trying to describe it and pointing at it, but she just thought I had smooth lost my mind. It was so funny!"

"Well, that will keep happening to you. Sometimes it is really frustrating," said Marie. "You just can't come up with the right word, even though it is on the tip of your tongue."

"Abby e-mailed me this week. Said she is doing fine, the meds are working better and better. She is getting ready to go back to school and looking forward to it. She said to tell everyone 'hi' and especially you, Carleton," said Marie.

"I miss her," said Carleton.

"I think we all do. She was so positive, when she was waiting for the meds to start working," said Missy.

"Missy, I know it is hard right now, but your meds are going to start working, too, and you're going to start feeling a lot better. I told you it took me five years to find the right meds; it doesn't take nearly as long now. They have so many more meds and they work much better. You're going to be fine," said Marie. Marie twisted a hank of her hair around her finger.

"I think so, too," said Carleton. "I do well with lithium, and it is the only med I have to take, other than a couple of supplementals. It's cheap and I don't have any side effects with it."

"I hope you guys are right," said Missy, "it's hard to be patient."

"Didn't you know that is the last thing a person with bipolar has—patience? We all have that in common."

"I haven't told you all, but my DWI case comes up this week. I'm scared to death," said Missy.

"Did you get the letter from the doctor for the judge?" asked Carleton

"Yes, and he wrote me a really good one, saying that I wasn't drinking anymore and I was working hard on getting traction with my bipolar, keeping my appointments and taking my meds."

"That sounds good. I don't think you have much to worry about. I know it is scary to go to court on something like this, but you actually have a defense. How many people have a defense for DWI?" said Marie.

"I think you are going to be fine," said Suzy.

"I wish I could be so confident," said Missy.

"Missy, you are going to do fine in court. Let me tell you, wear a skirt, not pants. I used to work in the courts and judges like that. Give him your letter and don't say anything, just answer his questions. As for your medications,' said Marie, "I'm looking forward to next week to and how much better you will be."

Chapter Twenty-Seven

Everyone was already sitting around the big table at Denny's when Missy walked in.

"Hey, everybody, here's Missy! How did it go at court?" asked Carleton.

"Much better than I thought it would," said Missy, with a big smile. She signaled the waitress to being her a Diet Coke.

"I can't believe how well it went. The judge read my doctor's letter and went for it. He sentenced me to a year's probation, no fine, and if I don't get into any trouble for a year, I get my license back and the DWI goes off my record," said Missy.

"That's great, said Marie, "it couldn't have gone any better."

"I'm happy for you," said Suzy.

"It'll be great to get your license back. I don't have one anymore and it is a pain to have to take the bus everywhere," said Carleton.

"I'm really happy," said Missy.

Jackie said, "You forgot to ask how it went for me at court last week."

"That's right, you weren't here last week. You were in court?" asked Marie.

"Yes, I asked for a custody hearing. It was really informal because I can't afford a lawyer, but I think I made progress. I told the judge my plans, and he said that if I go to school this fall and do well, I could start having David on weekends. Then we'll see how that goes."

"Jackie, that is wonderful," said Marie, "why didn't you tell us you were going to court?

"I guess I was a little superstitious, thinking it would go badly if I talked about it. It went well, all considering. I just can't believe I have to fight my own parents for my child."

"I know," said Missy "that's the pits. However, you are making progress. From what you told us, you were just lying on the couch for a couple of years, and now you are planning on going back to school and working to get custody of David back."

"Yes, hasn't she done well?" said Suzy. "I'm inspired by her and trying to do as well as she does, but missing Manny seems to hold me back."

"Well, try not to think of him all the time," said Marie.

"How can I do that? I really love him and miss him. I don't think I want to stop thinking about him," said Suzy.

"It's too much to ask of her," said Jackie, "it's too hard."

"Suzy, you are obsessed with him and you need to tell your doctor. You are never going to move ahead if you don't get past this," said Marie. "Remember how obsessed Abby was and how quickly her meds helped?"

"Yeah, Suzy, you really need to work on that. It's all you ever talk about," said Missy.

Suzy blew up. "I told you I am NOT obsessed! I just miss him is all. Knowing how much he loved me and how much I missed by being excluded from the last months of his life has made me sad." Suzy started crying now. "There is a big difference between being sad and being obsessed and I am not obsessed. Jackie understands, and if any of the rest of you cared about me, you would understand, too. I am not going to stay here and be insulted like this."

"Suzy, my husband died two years ago, and while I still miss him, I don't talk about him all the time. It would bore you silly to constantly hear me talk on the subject. I am not obsessed, just sad. It is you who act obsessed," said Marie.

Suzy stood and stalked out of the restaurant. Jackie said, "I'll go with her and try to talk to her."

"I am sorry she is upset but she is never going to get off square one if she doesn't work on that. Maybe we should have upset her earlier," said Marie.

"I know how easy it is to have your feelings hurt when you are not stable. What about your husband?" Missy asked.

"I don't want to talk about it right now, with Suzy so upset," said Marie. She started to twist a piece of hair around her finger.

"And now to my problem," said Carleton.

"What are you having problems with, Carleton?" asked Marie.

"There was some difficulty at the clinic this week, don't ask me what, and they couldn't give me my lithium prescription."

"Do you need lithium? I can mail you some this afternoon because I have some just lying around my medicine cabinet. I took it for a while. They tried me on it first just to see if I would respond to it. " said Missy.

"No, I have a stash that will last me for a week or two until they get this straightened out. Of course, they don't know about that. And if all else fails, I'll get some lithium batteries, grind them up, and snort them."

Everyone laughed at that.

"Of course we have to take every chance to get ahead on your meds because they are always screwing up on your prescriptions or for some reason you can't get the scrip filled. I never tell them when I get ahead for fear they'll cut back on my meds and I'll be unable to get them at some point. I guess that's why we all have these extra meds," said Marie. "They want us to have only and exactly what we need, so we can't overdose, but that is taking the chance of running out due to some unforeseen circumstance."

"For us it's a real emergency not to have our meds, to them it means nothing. It means a trip to the emergency room for us; it's inconvenient for them to put themselves out to make sure we always have them when we need them. Just can't do without them," said Carleton.

"I've never missed a doctor's appointment in twenty-five years and I hate to think what would happen if I got sick or my car broke down or something. They always say that if you skip an appointment you won't get your meds. So your punishment for being sick is going crazy," said Marie.

Just then, Suzy and Jackie returned. Suzy's eyes were red, but she was calm.

"Suzy, I'm sorry we upset you. I really think you should talk about this with your doctor, said Marie.

"And I have to agree with that," said Missy.

"I have told Suzy that it can't do her any harm to discuss these thoughts with her doctor, and Suzy has agreed," said Jackie.

"As I told you, I don't think I am obsessed, and I am going to prove it to you by telling my doctor about the thoughts I have about Manny and see what she thinks," Suzy said.

"Suzy, if you can prove us wrong, you will make us happy and we'll be happy to shut up about it. We just worry about you and want you to get better," said Marie.

"Yes," said Missy. "We aren't trying to make life hard on you; we are trying to help."

"It is hard for me, but I will talk to the doctor about it and see what she says."

"Thanks, Suzy," said Marie.

"We were just talking about the consequences we all face if we can't get our meds," said Carleton.

"Like if you go crazy 'cause you can't get your meds, you go to jail instead of to the hospital. Hospitals are bad enough, Jackie, but it is no fun to go to jail when you are manic," said Carleton.

"Have any of you read Pete Earley's book, *Crazy*? Now that is really good," said Marie.

"Can I get it at the library?" asked Suzy.

"Sure, it's really good, about how mentally ill people are treated in this country."

"I'll have to get a copy," said Jackie

"I think I know enough already," said Carleton.

"It's just so frustrating how we are treated. I lost the job I had for nine years just because I had bipolar disorder. Everything was fine until they found out I was nuts, then I couldn't work there anymore," said Marie. "They seemed to think I was going to shoot up the place any minute."

"I know; the stigma is terrible. I can't even raise my own child," said Jackie.

"We need some civil rights for crazy people, some inalienable rights for nutcases," said Carleton.

"You are right, Carleton," said Marie, "but don't hold your breath."

"You remember Andrea Yates, the one who drowned her five children?" said Marie.

"Oh, yes," said Suzy.

"Right," said Missy.

"Oh yeah, I remember that one," said Jackie.

"Well, she was just as psychotic as they come, and in her first trial they convicted her of murder even though it was obvious she was insane," said Marie.

"Yes, they always want to punish mentally ill people," said Missy.

"It makes me want to give up sometimes, but of course that is what bipolar people do—give up. Did you know that twenty-five percent attempt to kill themselves? And sixteen percent succeed," Marie said.

"I know it is hard to get diagnosed, to get help, to get any kind of understanding. Well, at least all of us are on the road to becoming stable," said Missy.

"Yes, said Jackie, you have to fight for it, but you can get better if you work on it."

"You're forgetting something, you know. Bipolar disorder has some good aspects," said Carleton.

"What is it you like, Carleton, the overspending binges or the hyper-sexuality?" asked Marie.

"I'm not talking about that, I mean the positive aspects. You know that many creative people were and are bipolar. You can name many famous people with bipolar disorder."

"You are right, there is that extra spark of creativity that so many of us seem to get: Vincent Van Gogh, Louisa May Alcott, Patty Duke, Carrie Fisher, and so many more. And don't forget, Winston Churchill," said Marie.

"Winston Churchill?" asked Jackie.

"Yes, as he has become less of an iconic figure and more of a regular human, it has been reported that he, too, had bipolar disorder. It is said that he had many, many ideas and it was his aides' job to decide which ones were good," said Marie. "Somehow, and luckily, he managed to go through the entire Second World War, working twenty hours a day, without his mood dipping into depression."

"I knew that a lot of people who were bipolar were extra creative, but I would not have thought of Winston Churchill as one of them," said Carleton.

"You probably have that spark of genius, Carleton, in your music, but I am afraid it has passed me by," said Marie.

"You never know what will happen, Marie."

"Missy, are you feeling any better this week?" asked Marie.

"Going to court took a great weight off my mind, and I think the meds are helping some, but I still don't feel stable."

"Keep working at it. You'll start to feel better. I know it is hard, but you can do it. You can always call any of us during the week if you need someone to talk to," said Marie.

"Boy, we talked a lot this week. Wonder if we will have that much to talk about next week?"

"Wait a minute. In terms of eating, I thought of something that is easy to fix and tastes good, like we were talking about a couple of weeks ago. How about—taquitos!"

"Oh great, now you will have all of us eating them," said Missy.

"Yes, those sound good," said Jackie.

"I know I'm going to the grocery store this afternoon," said Suzy.

As they all left, Marie called out to Missy, "Hey, wait for me."

Missy stopped and turned around, looking quizzically at her. "What's up?"

When Marie caught up with her, she said, quietly, "I want to drive you home today. I don't want you waiting for the bus in this heat."

"Great! I'll go along with that."

They slowed down a little, waiting for the others to leave. Then they got in Marie's car and headed out. "Why did you want to take me home?" Missy asked.

"I wanted to ask how you were doing with your latest meds, and I really don't like it that you have such a long bus ride. It is so hot."

"As for my meds, they don't seem to be working so well. The doc says as soon as I get weaned off these he will start me on some new ones. I just can't seem to find the right ones."

"Oh, I know how frustrated you are. I tried for so long and it seemed like I would never get there. However, I did, and I have been on good medications for years. I can't tell you what a difference it makes. Please keep trying, even though I know it isn't easy."

"I will, but it is really hard. Hey, could you stop at that drugstore on the corner? I need to get something."

Marie pulled into a parking place and Missy got out of the car and walked rapidly into the store without looking back. She was inside only a few minutes; Marie was just starting to get uncomfortably warm when she reappeared.

Missy got back in the car. She had a small sack in her hand. She didn't say anything. Marie stared at the sack. "Oh, I guess I'll tell you since you drove me here. It's a pregnancy test."

"For God's sake…"

"I know, I know, I should have been more careful. It was stupid of me and now I don't know what I'll do if I am pregnant."

Marie started the car and drove towards Missy's mother's house. "Please call me tonight after you take the test if it is positive. I will come right over and we'll figure things out. Promise?"

"Okay, I will. I just hope I'm not."

"I hope so too. Call me if you need me."

"Okay, I will," said Missy, as she got out of the car.

Marie drove home, upset, and then didn't leave her place all evening. She mostly just paced around, waiting for the phone to ring. She finally went to sleep, late, when it didn't.

Chapter Twenty-Eight

When they were all assembled the next week, Missy's face lit up and she said, "You all are not going to believe what happened this week!"

Marie held her breath.

"What?" ..."What happened?" ..."I'll bet you're going to tell us," they all chorused.

"Let's get our food and Cokes first."

Everyone waited impatiently until all the food and drinks were sorted out.

"You just won't believe it—I got my Social Security!"

Marie's whole body relaxed.

"Already? That is hard to believe. That's the fastest I ever heard of anyone getting it," said Marie.

"Mine was much faster, but I think Missy has set a record," said Suzy.

"I got mine in a matter of months, but it's only been weeks for you, Missy," said Jackie.

"I got my SSI really fast, too," said Carleton.

I have income now," Missy said, "and the first thing I am going to do is to move into my own apartment. My mother helped me out a lot by taking me in after I lost my apartment, my car, my furniture, just everything, but that doesn't keep her from driving me nuts."

"I know, it's much better on your own," said Marie.

"I stayed with my parents longer than I should have, but that was because of David," said Jackie.

"I was lucky. My parents paid for my house, so I could have a place of my own," said Suzy.

"And I've been on my own for years," said Carleton. "Sometimes it gets lonely. That's when wish I could have a cat. How is Charlie doing, anyway?"

"He's doing much better. He only asks to go out early in the morning and evening now. My neighbors have not reported him being loose because they are all crazy about him," said Marie. "Yesterday I was so worried about him— I let him out about 6:00 a.m. and by 9:00 he wasn't back. That was unusual. I looked, waited, and got all anxious. I finally found him asleep in the laundry basket I keep in the bathroom. He had used the cat door and I hadn't heard him. That was a relief."

"What do you do all day?" asked Suzy." We can't go shopping because none of us have the money"

"Yeah. I just go to the grocery store and if I need anything else, I go to Wal-Mart," said Jackie.

"I spend most of my day reading and sometimes I write a little, and I watch a little TV," said Marie.

"What shows do you watch?" asked Suzy. "You already said that you don't watch the late shows."

"I like *Dateline* and *20/20* and *Sixty Minutes* and a couple of the talk shows; I don't like fictional shows. Of course, I watch *Jeopardy*.

"So you must like Reality shows," said Missy.

"Lord no, those things aren't real. They are staged and scripted and most of them are real boring," said Marie.

The others laughingly agreed.

"Hey, I had a great idea for a reality show, and this one couldn't be scripted," said Suzy.

"What was it?"

"Well, you get twenty hard-core, unstable bipolars and you put them in a house together."

"This has possibilities," said Carleton.

"Some of them are paranoid, and think they are always being watched," Suzy explained.

"Sure," said Marie, "that would happen."

"A couple of them would be angry all the time and no one could speak to them without setting them off," said Suzy.

"That sounds right," said Jackie.

"The others would just cry and bitch and moan all time about how terrible their lives were," said Suzy.

"And one or two would go around comforting everyone and trying to be peacemakers, though they would have their rough patches, too," described Suzy. "Nobody could sleep at night, so everyone would be up all night, getting on each other's nerves and pissing everyone else off."

"Except two of them, who would sleep through the night and then play music all day and disturb everyone else," interjected Marie.

"Oh yes," said Carleton.

"And don't forget the hypersexual ones, who would be off in corners doing something inappropriate every chance they got, which would upset everyone else; but they wouldn't care and would just keep on doing it," said Marie.

"How would the free-spending ones mess things up?" said Carleton.

"I don't know," said Suzy, "maybe the TV channel would give everyone a credit card with a limit for necessities. The binge spenders would spend all their money on unnecessary, frivolous things like pastries and CDs, and then try to borrow cigarettes, shampoo, soap, and razor blades from the more responsible ones."

"Oh, this is fun, Suzy, but how does the game work?" said Jackie.

"That's simple. You get so many points for a meltdown, so many for a crying jag, so many for irritating a group of people. Yelling, bitching get points, but you have to leave the house if you become too disruptive. At the end of say, ten weeks, the person with the most points who is still in the house wins six month's medications and therapy in the best mental health hospital in the country."

"Wouldn't that be worth it?"

"I don't know Suzy, the therapy and meds sound good, but I don't know if I could take ten weeks surrounded by that many unstable bipolars," said Marie.

"It would be worth it to me," said Missy.

"Can you imagine how judgmental the American public would be watching something like this? Most of them don't even believe there is such a thing as mental illness," said Suzy.

It would be like watching those hoarder shows—you just can't believe what you are seeing. They would think it was scripted and wouldn't believe it was real!"

"They would have to pay everyone to get them to do it," said Jackie.

"I don't know," said Carleton. "Ten weeks of free room and board might be enough to attract unstable bipolars. It would get them out of their parent's houses."

"That would make everyone happy," said Missy.

Everyone laughed. "That's an interesting idea, Suzy. It strikes me as funny, but I think you would have to have bipolar disorder to get it and find it humorous," said Marie.

"Oh sure, the general public doesn't have a clue as to what the parameters of bipolar behavior are, so they would just sit there with their mouths open, unable to see that all the strange behavior is what we recognize as 'normal,'" said Jackie.

"I think we should pitch the idea. There are some twisted people in Los Angeles. They would think that the freak factor would garner a large audience and lots of advertisers. They wouldn't care what it did to the people in the house," said Carleton.

"You are probably right, Carleton, but I don't really think it would educate anyone. As you said, people would just watch it for the freak factor, as they do the hoarding shows, and they do not really grasp the problems of having bipolar disorder. It takes an insider to see the humor and predictability of it," said Marie. "On that note, I've got a doctor's appointment today, so I'll see you next week."

Chapter Twenty-Nine

Marie walked into Denny's the next Wednesday a little late. Things seemed a little off. No one wanted to start talking, so they ordered food and drinks and then, silence. Finally, Marie asked Suzy, "Did you go to the doctor?"

"Yes, I did. And you will not believe this, she is not certain that I am obsessed with Manny. She said there is a possibility that I am. To test it out, she is putting me on a new medication. So see, you were wrong."

"I am glad to be wrong if it means that you are okay."

"I asked you about your husband a while back and you didn't answer. Is that because you don't want to talk about him?" Missy asked.

"No, I don't mind talking about him. He and I were only married two years and were happy with each other, but he died suddenly from a heart attack. I moved to Dallas to get away from all the memories…. I miss him still," said Marie. She twisted a piece of hair in her fingers.

"Then you do know what it is like," said Suzy.

"I do. However, he disappointed me big time. He put his money in trust for his stepson and all I owned was my car and half of the house. I had to sell the house to get the money out of it; I had a good job so wasn't too worried. Then, I developed an allergy to my medication and I had to stop taking it. The doctor started me on a new one, which, unfortunately, was fraudulently sold as a treatment for bipolar when it really had no effect on it. Goddamn drug companies. Anyway, there I was, operating without sleep or stability and my boss was beginning to think I was a drug addict, so I actually told her that I had bipolar disorder. Well, you can imagine, that was the end of me. I looked and looked for a new job, but I guess I was too old."

"You had it rough," said Missy.

"No worse than any of the rest of you," said Marie. "Being bipolar just means you are going to have a hard time in this world. You aren't going to get a lot of help or sympathy along the way. Oh, I should tell you that my boss was an RN, so I thought I could tell her and she would understand. That didn't work."

"What was your job?" asked Suzy.

"I was a writer for a medical training company. I could only find one book about bipolar disorder when I was diagnosed. Of course, there are dozens now. I wish I had Patty Duke's to read when I needed it."

"Yes, her book is good, and there are many others. They are a help when you are feeling like you are struggling alone," said Jackie.

"And, of course, Kay Jamison is so inspiring. I guess we have all read her books," said Marie.

"No, I haven't," said Missy.

"Those are the ones you need to read. They will make you see it is possible to get stable and stay that way," said Marie.

"Okay, just let me write her name down so the next time I go to the bookstore I can look her books up. I want to read your book, too."

"You can get it from Amazon," said Marie.

"Missy, sometimes I forget how new you are to this. I wish I could help you more," said Marie.

"You all have helped me a lot. I just don't understand why I'm having such a hard time, and Abby took pills for six weeks and was completely straightened out."

"It is never the same for any two people. The disease is so individual. Some people try for years and never find medications that work. Most people respond to medications. However, you'll never be 'normal.' It's hereditary, so there is nothing you can do about it," said Marie.

"That's right—I never told you about my Aunt Blanche, did I?"

"No, you didn't."

"What about her?"

"My mother told me about her after I crashed. That's how she got me to the Mental Health Clinic. I never heard this stuff before. My Aunt Blanche would get manic, they didn't know that then, and run off from her husband and kids. Eventually she would crash and come home, but my uncle got tired of it and divorced her. Of course, he got custody of the kids.

She kept getting married, doing the same thing, and her husbands always gave up on her. Finally, after so many years, she hanged herself in her closet. Mom told me that story to get me to realize that what I was doing was really serious."

"Missy, that is awful. How scary. At least now we have some knowledge of the syndrome so doctors can treat it," said Jackie.

"Yes, it's only been a generation since they have been able to treat it, even though the ancient Greeks could diagnose it. No wonder they don't have the treatment down yet. We can only hope that it gets better as the years pass. I'm waiting for a blood test or a brain scan that will indicate what drugs I should take. Did you know they have a brain scan that can diagnose it now? It costs several thousand dollars and I am satisfied with my diagnosis, but it could be useful, as it gets cheaper. Now the doctor can only go by your behavior," said Marie.

"Missy, you don't want to underestimate the power of the stigma that accompanies the illness. You know that you have a disorder that messes with your mood and may cause you to do strange things, but the general public believes you are out of your mind," said Jackie.

"Yes," said Marie. "You want to confide in people, but be sure they won't hold it against you. Never tell an employer. When Jessie Jackson, Jr., announced his diagnosis, I read some of the comments to the news stories on the Internet. You wouldn't believe the things people said. It actually hurt my feelings. Some people said that he was actually a drug addict or an alcoholic. One person said that he was too crazy to remain in the House; another said that he should resign because he might lose control in the halls of Congress and start raping women. There is no general knowledge of the actual effects of the disorder on a person. To the man on the street, there is no difference between a person on medication and one who is not. People are afraid of those with bipolar disorder. It is depressing to see it written out like that."

"I have tried to fight against the stigma by writing my book, but some people who read it don't think I am describing it accurately. They review my book and say that I am not crazy enough to have bipolar disorder. It is really something you have to be careful about, but I guess all of us have had to learn it the hard way. Just don't get yourself hurt. Tell only family and close friends."

"That is depressing. I'm glad you told me this. I will be careful. When you are first diagnosed, you sort of want to tell everyone, so they'll know why you were acting so weird. I've only told family and you all. I'd better keep it that way. It's getting late. I'll see you guys next week," said Missy.

Chapter Thirty

The informal support group gathered the next week and after ordering drinks, salads, and some other foods, Jackie spoke up, "You know we have talked about so much—Social Security, my fight with my parents, Marie losing her husband, stigma, medications—but one thing we haven't talked about is Carleton. We have yet to hear his story."

"I am not so extraordinary," he answered. "It's just that even when I take my lithium like I'm supposed to, I still get manic on a regular basis, and then I usually lose my job and have to move."

"That sounds serious. What do you do?" said Suzy.

"I have a tendency to take off all my clothes and walk down the street, trying to give away money," said Carleton.

"Oh, boy, that must upset your neighbors," said Marie.

"Yes, they get scared and call the police, and I either go to jail or to the hospital. It doesn't matter; I'll be locked up either place. I get my lithium faster at the hospital."

"How do the cops take it?" asked Marie.

"They think it is funny," said Carleton.

"I thought as much. They aren't going to be frightened by something like that," said Marie.

"But it must be hard on you, Carleton," said Jackie.

"Yes, it completely screws up my life. The neighbors are afraid of me, and sometimes I am gone so long I lose all my belongings to an eviction. The people I work with and for are not that understanding and fire me. There is nothing I can do about it."

"That's awful," said Suzy.

"Sometimes I get discouraged because I can't get any traction. Even my friends desert me after one of my episodes. My sense of humor is the only thing that keeps me going. That, and my music," said Carleton.

"We'll never abandon, you, Carleton, we'll always be your friends. No matter what happens, we will be here for you," said Missy.

"Absolutely," said Jackie

"You can count on it, said Suzy.

"We're the six Musketeers. We'll always be together," said Marie.

Carleton began to sing the old song, "Stand by Me," interrupted by the others' laughter.

"You're counting Abby?" said Carleton.

"Of course, you know you can always e-mail her. If you need something. We haven't heard from her lately, but I know she is just getting ready to return to Virginia Tech. It is her fourth year, and I'll bet she is both excited and worried about it," said Marie.

"That does make me feel better," said Carleton. "I've wanted friends all my life, and now I have five. I feel like I can count on you guys. I enjoy so much talking with you and having these meetings with you. In some ways, these weeks have been happiest of my life."

Jackie added, "That is great. I think we all feel we haven't wasted our time if one of us feels that much better because of our meetings."

"I was feeling pretty friendless since I just moved down here. You are really the first people I have got close to. This has helped me come out of my shell since Brad died," said Marie.

I think we have all gained from the encouragement and way we have listened to each other," said Jackie.

"We are like 'flying buttresses,'" said Marie.

"Yes," exclaimed Carleton, as he slammed his hand down on the table.

Suzy nodded, but Jackie and Missy just looked puzzled.

Marie said, "You'll know just what I mean when I tell you what a flying buttress is. When they built the medieval Gothic cathedrals, the interiors were twelve stories tall, with the walls made of stained glass. When you walk into one, it looks like a miracle that it could stand. It is open, light, and airy and you can't see what supports the walls. But if you look from the outside, you'll see flying buttresses propping up the arches that hold up the walls and the ceiling. That's what we are, people who are propping each other up without the world knowing."

"Oh, that is a great image," said Jackie, with Missy saying at the same time, "I get it. We support each other, but unseen."

"That will be how we think of one another," said Jackie.

"And, Jackie, do you ever want to talk about your rape?" said Marie.

"When we first started, I didn't know you all well enough to talk much about it; now, after working with the therapist, I really don't feel the need to go into any detail with you. I know you all believe me that it actually happened, so I am okay with it. It has taken a long time, but I am putting it behind me. The thing that kept me from dealing with it was those who didn't believe me."

"That's the worst," said Marie.

"Yes, I don't know why people would disbelieve you." said Suzy.

"Speaking as a man, I would never have the nerve to say that I didn't believe what a woman said about that."

"It used to just infuriate me," Jackie said," but now I can take it more in stride. As you said, Marie, people are so ignorant about mental illness they assume that I would just make something up."

"I think we have all done better this summer," said Missy, "though I don't seem to be getting well as fast as I want to. This week I am having the weirdest sensation—I feel like there are bugs crawling up and down my legs. It's especially bad at night. I don't know what to do. It's driving me crazy."

Carleton said, "I know what it is; it's a side effect of one of the meds you are taking. It's called 'Restless Leg Syndrome' and you need to take a certain med for it. I know, because I have a similar problem. Go ahead and call your doctor or psychiatric nurse and she'll give you a prescription."

"Really? Oh, God, I thought I was going crazy for sure. Excuse me, you all."

Missy leaned over and pulled her purse from under the table. She reached in, grabbed her phone, and was able to dial her doctor from memory. She got the nurse right away. She described her symptoms and told her what Carleton said. She was on the phone for a few minutes, then turned back to the group and said,

"Thank you so much. She knew exactly what I was talking about and she is going to call the pharmacist right away. She says I'll be able to sleep tonight."

"Things aren't usually that easy to fix, but that went smoothly," said Marie.

Missy answered, "Yes, I wish you all could always tell me what to do."

"If we could, then we could all dispense with the rather annoying doctors we have to deal with," said Jackie.

"That would be nice," said Marie. "There have been times when I have known more about it than the doctors have. Not a lot of the time, though. You know, now there is a new treatment with magnets, but it only works for a few people, and of course, it is expensive. Isn't that weird—magnets. The dang thing is such a mystery. I will be so glad when they can nail it down. Don't know if it will happen in my lifetime, though. It doesn't seem like it, but they have made great progress since they first discovered that lithium would help. It just seems slow when you are in the middle of it."

"Especially, said Missy, "When you are waiting for your pills to work."

"That's the truth, you only have faith to sustain you then, and it is hard to believe that you will get better. But it will happen, we are all testaments to that," said Marie, "just keep plugging away and you'll get there."

"The doctor said that if I am not feeling better by next week, we'll try another drug; so at least I know he is still working on it," said Missy.

"Yes, it's just slow," said Jackie.

"You know, said Marie, some people confuse getting medication with medicating themselves, either with drugs or alcohol. Missy, I think you were doing that when you were drinking so much. Alcohol is a depressive, and you were so manic you were trying to bring yourself down with it."

"Really?" said Missy. "I never thought of it that way. But I'll bet you are right. I never drank like that before."

"I swear, celebrities have the worst of it. They live in a culture that is surrounded by drugs, and they try to self-medicate with drugs. They have access to the drugs, and people 'help' them out by making it easy for them to get them. Because they are well known and loved, they can create all kinds of havoc before they are stopped. Patty Duke's autobiography is a good example of that, as is Carrie Fisher's."

"Yeah, but regular people crash just as hard," said Jackie, "they just don't do it as publicly and usually they run out of resources faster. At the same time, they are likely to end up in jail rather than a psychiatric ward or a rehab facility."

"Some people don't believe that a person who is abusing drugs or alcohol is bipolar; they don't realize that is often the most visible symptom of the illness. Nobody gets through bipolar disorder without some destruction. We are bound to create some ruin as we reel toward diagnosis," said Carleton.

"I was lucky. I smoked marijuana for ten years to sleep, but never got addicted to anything but cigarettes, and God knows they were hard enough to quit," said Marie.

"Well, I drank enough alcohol that it is a wonder I am not dead," said Missy. "I feel a whole lot better since I stopped."

"We'll look forward to seeing how you feel next week," said Suzy.

Chapter Thirty-One

The group was sitting at their usual table at Denny's, quietly talking, except for Suzy. She pushed the door open and ran up to the table. She sat down and then spilled out, "I think I was obsessed with Manny. Since I have started on this new medication I don't hear his songs in my head and I don't think about him all the time."

"That's great," said Marie.

"It's a real win for you," said Missy, "and I am sure Abby would say so, too. You should e-mail her and tell her that you broke your obsession, too."

"I told her it would change her life," said Jackie.

"It already has, but it embarrasses me."

"There is nothing to be embarrassed about; it was just part of your illness. Now you have it under control with medication. It was certainly not your choice. I guess I do know what you mean. I have been embarrassed by things I did when I wasn't in control, also," said Marie.

"I know I have been there, too," said Carleton.

"Me, too, said Missy, throwing away everything I owned for a guy who didn't give a shit about me." She wiped away a tear.

"And I wrecked a perfectly good car for no good reason," said Jackie.

"I think that is one of the reasons we are talking, so we can get all that stupid stuff off our chests and go forward from here. I know we have all lost a lot of friends and relationships, but we just have to let it go. We can't change it; we just have to do better in the future," said Marie.

"But it is so hard to live with what you have done," said Missy.

Marie answered, "Yes, it is. However, we don't get do-overs. At least none of us spent money irrationally. Some people with bipolar can spend thousands of dollars on things they don't need and really don't want when they come down from their high. And they are stuck with paying for it or declaring bankruptcy."

"Well, I sort of had that problem—I gave up a paid-for car for a fancy new SUV that I couldn't pay for and lost. I let my boyfriend influence me," said Missy.

"Yes, that is one thing I'm glad to do without," said Jackie, "I did enough damage the way I was."

"I knew someone who ran up thirty thousand dollars on e-Bay in one evening. He had no way to pay it and didn't even want the items when he sobered up. You can't get out of debts by saying, 'I have bipolar disorder.' Doesn't work," said Marie. She continued, "I don't like the way they always convict people with bipolar disorder of crimes. They say that we know the difference between right and wrong so we are guilty. They don't take into account that we can't control our actions, so it is not always our fault. I would take back most of what I did if I could."

"So would we all," said Carleton." I'd still be working and I wouldn't have to move every time I got manic."

"Everybody gets something they have to deal with in their lifetime—we are just the lucky ones who got bipolar disorder. All we can do is try our best to find good doctors and insist on the best medications, and then take them regularly to remain stable. And read all we can about it so we can stay up with the newest research," said Marie.

"I have gained a lot coming to these meetings and talking about what's bothering me and what happened to me, but I am afraid this will be the last one for me. School starts soon and I have to get ready," said Jackie.

"So you are going back to school. I want to do that, too, when I get straight," said Missy.

"Where are you going to go?" asked Carleton.

"I'm starting out at Richland College, where I can get the basics out of the way, and then when I finish them I'll transfer to a four-year school to get my Bachelor's."

"Which college do you want to go to?" asked Suzy.

"I hope I don't ruin it for myself by telling you all, but I hope to do well enough to go to the University of Texas at Austin. I don't know what I am going to major in yet, but I think it will have something to do with writing."

"I think you will get in and you will do well. I used to teach in junior colleges in Oklahoma City and they give you a good background without costing so much," said Marie.

"I want to stay close to David, and at the same time I want to get a good degree so I can get a job and prove that I am capable of caring for him, so this seems like the best way to start," said Jackie.

"Jackie, I'll miss you like crazy, I've enjoyed hearing your stories and listening to your good sense for the past months. I just hope everything works out for you and that you gain custody of David. You are taking the right steps toward getting him back," said Marie. "Don't you all think so?"

"It sounds like a good plan to me," said Carleton. "Keep in touch with us through e-mail. I hope you get David back, soon."

"I will miss your encouragement and all the help you have given me," said Missy. "After hearing what you have been through, and seeing where you are now, I just know I will make it."

"I've come a long way, but you all have helped me, and I will miss you," said Jackie.

"This is kind of an awkward time to be telling you this, but this is my last time to come, too," said Suzy.

"Why, Suzy, have you got some plans, too?" asked Marie.

"Yes, I have been thinking about them for quite a while, but I just made the decision last week when I was talking with my sister."

"Well, what are you going to do?" asked Missy.

"I have decided to go back to school, too. First, I am going to take the LSAT this fall, and spend the next few months clearing out my house and moving to this neighborhood."

Carleton leaned over and said quietly to Marie, "what's the LSAT?'

Marie whispered back, "The law school exam."

"I hadn't told you about my house before, but it is a real mess. It is going to take me a long time to clean it up and get rid of the things I don't need. I don't want to think about moving until I have done that."

"Why are you going to move into this neighborhood?" asked Carleton.

"Because my dad said he would pay for me to go to SMU Law School; all I have to do is get in."

"Well, you can do that," said Marie.

"Sure," chimed in Missy.

"With both of you leaving at once, it will mean a big hole in our group. How will we get along?" said Marie.

"You will have more time and attention to pay to Missy, who needs it right now," said Suzy.

"Missy, I'd sure like to hang around and see you make a breakthrough, but I really need to get on with the next phase of my life," said Jackie.

"My sister has promised me that she will help me on the weekends during the fall and I can't pass that up. I am going to be working on the house every day," said Suzy.

"Good luck to both of you and please, please, keep in touch," said Marie.

Jackie and Suzy left together.

After they got out the door, Marie turned to Carleton and Missy and said, "Just as soon as Jackie said she was leaving, then Suzy said she was going, too."

"Yeah, those two are really close. I hope they both do well. I guess it's down to us three for next week," said Missy.

Chapter Thirty-Two

Carleton and Marie were already in the Denny's when Missy came in, looking a little forlorn. She came over and sat down; the waitress already knew to bring her a Diet Coke. "It's going to be kind of lonely, with just the three of us."

"I know," said Marie, "two of our flying buttresses have fallen away. I wonder if the rest of us can offer each other enough support. We'll just have to do the best we can. I wanted to tell you, though, I read the biography of Manny, Suzy's friend, and nowhere does it have a mention of Suzy, even though it is six hundred pages long and talks about dozens of his women friends."

"That's what I thought," said Missy.

"Hey, one good thing, with only three in the group, we can spend more time on you. I don't think we had been paying enough attention to you before, and now we'll be able to," said Marie.

"What do you mean?" asked Missy.

"Most everyone else was pretty much stabilized, but you still need help and encouragement. I know you must be disheartened by the fact that it is taking so long for you to get traction with your meds," said Marie.

"I am, and sometimes I don't think I'll ever get there, but you all have spent a lot of time trying to get me to see I'll eventually get there. I want to ask you, though, about natural remedies," said Missy.

"No," said Carleton, "don't even think about it. Those aren't good."

"What do you mean?" asked Missy.

"They are just a way of separating you from your money and they don't give good results. You'll see people online saying how good they are, but they probably started taking them then reached a basic stable time or plateau between highs and lows, and they think it is the natural cure that has made them feel better. When they go manic or depressed again, they'll realize it was not the cure that did it, just the cycle, but it may be years between cycles for some people, so they aren't being protected against the next cycle. The only way to do that is to get on medication and stay on it."

"One guy sells pig food and calls it a natural supplement. I'm not kidding," said Carleton, "and he charges a lot for it."

"It's just as effective as taking natural remedies for heart disease, which I hope you would never do," said Marie. "It is a mental illness, but it has a physical cause and needs to be treated physically with medication."

"On another subject, you know what I think you should do? I think you should consider carefully before you fall in love again. Now, don't look at me that way. I'm bipolar, too, and I had plenty of bad relationships before I fell in love with Brad and married him. From what you've told us about your last guy—well, he was a real loser. How many guys have two babies they are supporting while they are professing to love someone else?" said Marie.

"Well, I was manic at the time and I don't think I was making good decisions. You know, I am bipolar," said Missy, with a lilt of sarcasm.

"I know that, Missy, but I guess what I really mean is that you probably shouldn't date anyone until you are stable. I know you are lonely and that it is hard to be alone, but you can't pick a good guy as long as you are subject to mania or depression." Marie frantically twisted a hank of hair.

"She's right," said Carleton, "you can't do anything that involves your emotions while you are unstable, but I think Marie is preaching to you and you don't need that."

"No, I sure don't." said Missy.

"I'm sorry; I didn't mean to sound like that. I am just trying to give you some advice that comes from my own life experience," said Marie.

"You sure make it sound easy," said Missy, "just get on the medication and everything will be all right. Well, I've been on medications for months and nothing is improving. I listen to all of you and you have it figured out, but I am out in the cold."

"Nobody is excluding you. I know it's easy to feel that way, but it is the illness talking," said Carleton.

"I felt like I could give you advice, because I thought we were so close. I know it sounds like I think I know a lot more than you do, but actually I have been diagnosed longer and I'm older. I told you about the guy I went with for ten years who ran around on me constantly, never took me out, and finally just walked out without saying 'good-bye.' That's the kind of man I chose before I got stable. So I am not criticizing you, I am just trying to get you to see that you should take it easy before you start on another relationship," said Marie, grasping a small lock of her hair and pulling it between her fingers.

"What makes you think I am about to have a relationship?"

"Both Carleton and I have noticed for the last two weeks you were driven here by a nice-looking young man," said Marie.

"So you are spying on me now?"

"No!" said Carleton. "We just happened to notice it. We thought you would tell us who he is, and when you didn't, we wondered if you didn't want us to know."

"I just wasn't ready to introduce him yet, is all. Don't I have a right to a private life?"

"Of course you do. I shouldn't have said anything. I just care so much about you, Missy."

Carleton chuckled, "Shit, neither of us has anything at all interesting about our lives, so we had to pay attention to yours. We'd have nothing to talk about if it weren't for you."

Missy laughed and relaxed. Marie felt uncomfortable that she had seemingly pushed Missy, and changed to a subject that she thought would be neutral.

She slipped the lock of hair neatly behind her ear and said, "I'll bet you are getting along with your mother a lot better since you moved into your own place,' said Marie.

"Yes, we are doing better, but mom still thinks I am going to go all 'Aunt Blanche' on her. Nobody trusts me to do anything right. I can't pick a man; I can't be trusted to run my own life. Look, my ride is here. I'll see you all next week." Missy walked rapidly out of the restaurant, without a backward look.

Marie said, "Oh, Jeez, Carleton, I don't think I could have screwed that up so badly if I had tried. I didn't mean to hurt her feelings. I just saw her with that guy and got scared for her."

"I know you were trying to help, but you came on pretty strong. Sometimes it's hard to remember how a person thinks when they are not stable," said Carleton.

"I acted like an idiot. She'll never listen to me again. I feel so bad, said Marie.

"We'll make it up to her next week. Maybe buy her a chocolate shake. Could be her medications might have kicked by then," said Carleton.

"I hope so. I so want her to feel better. I'll see you next week."

Chapter Thirty-Three

The next week, Carleton and Marie were at Denny's ahead of Missy. They had their drinks and sat so they could see the door. Marie asked Carleton, "how was your week?"

"It was normal; I went to the doctor and got my lithium. We had a gig Saturday night, and I enjoyed that. I especially enjoyed the extra money."

"Where did you play?"

"It was at the Adolphus Hotel, for a group of doctors."

"Oh, that must have been boring."

"Wasn't bad."

"You know, Missy has never been this late before."

"Probably got caught up with that guy."

"Oh, I hope not. I hate seeing her get involved with someone when she is not ready."

"Is anyone ever ready?"

"True, though I certainly did better after I got on my medication and got some stability going."

"I hope nothing has happened to her."

"No, she's just late; she'll be here in a minute."

"Since we have to wait, I guess I'll have some food, though I usually don't. I try not to gain any weight."

"What are you going to have?"

"Just a salad—do you want anything?"

Marie gestured to the waitress and when she came over, ordered a small salad. While she waited, she kept her eyes on the door.

"Watching the door isn't going to make her come any faster," said Carleton.

Marie laughed. "I know, but I am getting anxious. Oh, wait, isn't that her boyfriend's car?"

"No, his is newer."

"Carleton, I want you to shoot me if I start preaching to her like I did last week. That was a really stupid move."

"I know what you were trying to do—it's just that she is not stable now and everything you say to her sounds like criticism. It's hard to remember how you were when you weren't stable, but I know my feelings got hurt and I was quite combative when I was not feeling right. You'll just have to be patient with her until her meds start to work."

"You are right. I'll be more patient with her. I should understand if anyone does. I went for five years on medication that didn't work. I'll be the very epitome of patience, you'll see. Well, I am going to call her and see if she is coming."

Marie got her phone from her purse and called Missy's number. She got no answer; the phone just went to voicemail. Marie left a message for Missy to call if she weren't coming to the meeting. "I guess she is on her way, she doesn't answer."

"She ought to be here soon," said Carleton.

"This is making me nervous, I can hardly eat. I'm worried about her." Marie twisted her hair through her fingers. "She is not at all stable, you know."

"She's okay."

"Then why isn't she here?"

"Good Lord! You know how the traffic is. She probably got stuck at a broken light or something. This is Dallas, after all."

"Yeah, you're right. I shouldn't worry. But I am going to call again,"

Marie called Missy's number again, and again got no answer.

"It's been nearly an hour. She would have called us if she were all right. I'm going to call the police."

"It is odd that she hasn't called."

Marie called 911 and asked for someone to check on Missy. She gave the person who answered Missy's address and stated that she was late for a meeting with no explanation. She and Carleton had to wait about a half-hour before the patrolman called her back. He reported that Missy was home and there was nothing wrong with her.

"She just said to tell you she didn't want to see or talk to you again. Just leave her alone."

Marie said, "Are you sure that's what she said?"

The patrolman said, "Yes, she was quite definite."

"Thank you," said Marie.

As soon as she hung up the phone, Marie began to cry. Carleton asked. "What did he say?"

Marie blubbered, "He said she doesn't ever want to see us or talk to us again, Carleton, I just can't stand it. I like her and I was depending on her so much to be a friend. I am going to miss her so much!"

"We can still get together."

"No, I don't want to if Missy is not going to be here. Nothing against you, but you don't need me for anything. I wanted to help Missy get straight and find her way. I'm going to leave now, good-bye, Carleton."

With that, Marie stumbled out of the restaurant, eyes streaming with tears, and got in her car. She sat for a few moments, composing herself, and then drove off. Carleton paid her forgotten bill and left by himself.

Abby

Chapter Thirty-Four

Abby felt so relieved when she realized her medication was working. She found herself interested in life again, able to enjoy everyday happenings, and not obsessing about Philippe, what he was doing and thinking all the time. In fact, she found herself not caring about anything he might be involved with anymore. She didn't worry if he had found someone to take her place, or if he still thought about her. She also no longer had the urge to return to France to see him. It was a good feeling.

Abby didn't want to talk about it anymore. As far as she was concerned, the entire thing was over. She had bipolar disorder, she recognized that, and all she had to do was to stay on her medication to remain stable. That was the end of it.

When Sandy got home from work, Abby asked her, "What should I do about leaving my support group? They gave me a lot of help, but I really don't need anything else from them. All I really want to do is to get home, tell my parents what happened, and get ready for school to start." Abby had been talking to Sandy about the whole process as she got diagnosed and started taking her medication.

"Just stop by and tell them that you are okay, and that you are headed home. They will understand. They know what it feels like."

"Okay, that's what I'll do. I am anxious to talk with my parents. I owe them an explanation as to why I found it necessary to spend the summer with you instead of staying home and working. I appreciate you letting me stay here and your help in getting me to the Mental Health Center. I would still be wandering around wishing I knew what was wrong with me if it weren't for you."

"I am just glad I could help you. So many people have such a hard time getting diagnosed. You are lucky to have found a medication that works for you so fast. Many people are not that lucky and it takes them a long time to get straightened out. Are you thinking about leaving right away? Have you got reservations for the plane?"

"Yes, I'm good for the day after tomorrow. I'll stop by Denny's tomorrow and talk to the group. This will really surprise them."

Abby spent that evening taking Sandy out to a nice place for dinner and to a play. She was grateful to her and wanted to show her that she knew how much Sandy had done for her. "Sandy, I will never forget what you did for me. I'll always be your friend, and I will always be there for you if you need me. I can't express my thanks enough."

"I did no more for you than you would have done for me. I just happened to know what you needed. I'm so glad it worked out for you. Let me know how you get on and keep me updated on school. I'll miss you."

The next day, Abby went by Denny's, anticipating telling her friends the good news after they had given their greetings and were ready to talk. "I have an announcement to make. It is good news, though. My meds kicked in two days ago. That awful anxiety went away and I am no longer obsessing about the guy in France. In fact, I don't think about him anymore. I have no desire to go back to France and see him now. You have no idea what freedom that is. I was so anxious and so torn-up about him I just couldn't stay with my parents. They were trying so hard to make me feel better it was driving me nuts so I came out here to stay with my ex-roommate. She encouraged me to go to the Mental Health Center and you guys encouraged me to stay with it. I am going back to school at Virginia Tech and I want to spend a little time with my folks before I do. My flight to Connecticut leaves tomorrow morning."

Everyone congratulated her; Marie said, "I can't believe your med worked for you so fast—that is almost unheard of. I am so happy for you. I hope everything works out."

They all chorused "good-bye" and their hopes for a good school year to an excited Abby.

On the plane to Connecticut, Abby was so pumped up she couldn't keep her mind on the book she was supposed to be reading. She was not only looking forward to seeing her parents again, but she was also anxious about how they would take what she had to tell them. She sat in the back of the plane, her dark hair a curtain in the side of her face, which was inscrutable as she pretended to read the book. She didn't want to talk to any of her fellow passengers, as excited as she was; she just wanted to explain everything that had happened to her parents.

In her phone calls home, she just told them about the fun she was having with Sandy, and about the weather they were having in Dallas, which she considered unusual. She noted that the natives were unfazed by it. She had not confided in them about Philippe, or her obsession with him, or her diagnosis with bipolar disorder. She wanted to clear the air with them and get it all on the table before her fourth year of vet school.

After the plane landed, Abby tripped down the ramp, anticipating seeing her parents. There they were, waiting for her, but looking a little anxious. Her father swept her into a big hug, and her mother cried a little. All the way home, Abby chattered about the summer in Dallas, the people she met and the places she went. When they got home, she turned serious and asked her parents for a talk. "We can talk tomorrow if you are too tired tonight, but there are some things I need to tell you before I head off to school."

Abby's mother said, "We have known that there was something going on since you first came home from France; we just didn't know what was bothering you or how we could bring it up. I would be happiest talking it over tonight. I have been so worried about you. Let me put on some coffee and get out the coffee cake I made you. I know you like it."

"Oh, Mom, I really do. You shouldn't have gone to all that trouble."

"We are so happy to have you back home, and now we are going to find out what's been going on. You know, we have been worried about you, but we were waiting for you to tell us what was happening."

"Some of it is a little rough. I want to prepare you for that. When I was in Lyons, I fell in love with one of my professors, which wasn't smart. It was even dumber that he was married. I got really involved with him and then, when he didn't break up with his wife like he told me he would, I came home to get over him."

"Abby, that's awful. I knew something was bothering you, but you didn't want to talk about it," said her mother.

"No, because I was having this strange reaction. I couldn't get him out of my mind, I thought about him all the time, and I couldn't let go of him. I didn't want to worry you about it, so I went to stay with Sandy, hoping that I would just get over him. However, it didn't work that way; it just kept getting worse. Not only was he all I could think about, but time became resoundingly slow. I couldn't sleep at night as I thought the nights would never end. They just went on and on, and all I wanted was to get back to Phillippe. The days were not any better. They dragged out, filled with yearning, and all I wanted to do was to get to the end of the day so I could go to bed."

"You have really had it rough," said her father.

"Abby, were you pregnant?" asked her mother.

"No, nothing like that; I didn't mean to scare you."

"What happened was, Sandy knew enough about bipolar disorder to think that I should check it out at the Mental Health Center. Since I didn't know what else to do and I wasn't getting any better, I did. The doctor diagnosed me with it."

"Abby, I'm so sorry that you had to go through that by yourself," said her father.

Her mother had started to cry again.

"Hey, you guys, it's not as bad as it sounds. I had Sandy to help me understand, and a good doctor, and I met a group of people who were also bipolar who talked with me and explained a lot of what was going on to me."

"I was lucky. I got diagnosed, I had people to help, and the medication took hold right away. My symptoms are taken care of. I no longer care about that dude in France and I am ready to go into my fourth year with no problems."

"I don't really understand, dear. What is bipolar disorder?" said her mother.

"I knew that would be your first question. It is a mood disorder—a mental illness that affects your emotions rather than your thinking. I brought you a couple of books I picked out for you that will help you grasp it. Now, just be happy for me."

"I'm still worried sick about you," said her mother.

"Mother, you will understand so much more when you read the books and you won't be so anxious anymore."

Abby's parents read the books, switching when they were finished so each of them could read both of them. They had dozens of questions for Abby, and she answered all that she could. Slowly, they caught on to what she was going through and what her health problems were.

At first, they were reluctant to encourage her to go back to school in the fall, but she convinced them she could handle it. "Really," she assured them," my symptoms are controlled, and my thinking is clear. It was my mood that was out of whack; that was keeping me from operating correctly. You've been around me for the past couple of weeks—you can tell I am all right."

"I must admit," said her father, "you seem to be perfectly normal. It's hard for me to believe that there was anything wrong with you."

Abby went back to school and melded seamlessly into the life of the campus. She wasn't as perfectionistic as she was in the past, and found that making good grades was even easier than it used to be. Everything seemed to come to her more easily now.

In April, her professor suddenly entered the lab and told the class that a shooter had started raking the campus with gunfire. "Since we are in a different area, we are probably safe, but we want everyone to return to your homes and wait for an all-clear."

As the news spread across the country, Abby started receiving emails from the members of her support group back in Dallas, but she was able to assure them that she was fine, though shaken. She followed the story as compulsively as any student did. She shuddered as she learned about the man who shot up the campus and the severity of his mental illness. At least, she thought, if she were going to have a mental illness, it was something she could manage with attention and medication.

The next month she graduated with honors, her parents looking on with pride. They worried about her all year, thinking that she could not manage the stress, but she proved them wrong, and they were pleased she had.

After graduation, Abby interviewed with a veterinarian who specialized in horses in Virginia, where she could easily travel home for weekends and vacations. The vet she interviewed with asked, "Why did you study in France?"

Abby answered, "I had the opportunity to and I thought going to the oldest veterinary school in France and immersing myself in a different culture would be a positive experience."

"And was it?"

"Oh, yes. I learned so much. And not just about vet practice, but about how others live and think."

The doctor seemed impressed by her grades and honors at Virginia Tech and hired her right away. She celebrated by buying herself a couple of Labrador retriever pups.

Abby found a psychiatrist in town and took her medication faithfully. She hardly even thought of being bipolar—it was just a part of her, like so many other parts.

Suzy

Chapter Thirty-Five

S uzy was really nervous about the LSAT, but her sister explained the whole thing to her and assured her that she could do it. When it came time to actually take the test, Suzy didn't think it was so hard, though she would have to wait some weeks to find out how she did. Meanwhile she and Martha, her sister, tackled the house. It was one hot mess and needed a tremendous amount of work. Martha couldn't spend much time at it, but she encouraged Suzy and checked on her to make certain that she wasn't getting bogged down. She and Martha worked out a plan. Suzy would clean up one room at a time, working her way through the house until she had cleaned it all up. They knew it would take months to go through the accumulation, but Suzy had five months before the next semester started and she could pace herself.

"I swear, Suzy, I think you have saved every single book you have ever read, and that includes school textbooks," said Martha.

"To tell you the truth, I think I have. It will be hard for me to discard them now, but I know I have to cut my possessions down so I can move into an apartment close to school, and I need to clear this house out so Dad can sell it. He bought it for me and I owe him that."

"The one good thing about books is that I don't have to throw them in the dumpster—I can give them to the library and they will either keep or sell them. I don't have to feel like they are just going to be discarded. That makes me feel better about getting them out of the house," said Suzy.

"Are you not going back to speak with your group anymore?" asked Martha.

"No, they gave me some good advice and listened to me when I needed it, but since Jackie dropped out I really didn't feel like going back anymore. No one but Jackie was a real friend to me, though I liked them all. They are the ones who convinced me to get on with my life. And that's what I am doing."

"I'll call in the evenings and see how you are doing, and on Saturday mornings I'll come over and help. If you get bogged down let me know and I'll try to help redirect you," said Martha.

"Okay," said Suzy, "I'll talk to you later."

After Martha left, Suzy walked through the house. In some places it was hard to walk, but mostly it was books and objects piled on tables and chairs. Just by looking at them, Suzy could tell they were worthless and needed to be thrown out, but the job looked so immense she didn't know where or how to start. She went back to her den and sat in front of the television, watching CNN until her guilt moved her into the kitchen. There she encountered the store of garbage bags and cleaning supplies that Martha had brought over.

She thought of their plan, and decided to start in the back bedroom, a room she hardly ever went into. She had mostly forgotten she owned a lot of the things that were in this room. There were some tools, which she never used, and the closet was filled with clothing and shoes she hadn't worn in years.

There was a lot of stuff, but this room wasn't going to be so hard. She started hauling it out to the back door, and piled it up on the back porch. That first day she managed to get half of it outside and ready for Goodwill. Even she realized that the stuff was just nearly worthless, but it was hard to give it away. Somehow, it seemed a part of her.

Suzy was tired that night but felt like she had made some progress. The next day, she spent all day sorting and dragging things out to the back porch. She called Goodwill, told them she had some things to donate, and set a time for them to pick them up.

Then she called her father. "Hey, I'm just cleaning out the house so I can move and I found a bunch of tools. They are scheduled to go to Goodwill, but I thought you might want to come over and check them out before I let them go."

"I don't think I need any of them, but I'll come by in the morning and see what you've got. Around nine."

"Okay, see you then."

When her father came the next morning, she didn't hear him knock because she was working in the back of the house. He came around back and started inspecting the tools on the porch. She saw him there and came out.

"What do you think?"

"I can use a few of these, but most of them need to go to Goodwill. They can sell them and get some good out of them. How are you doing in the house?"

Suzy took him in to the back bedroom and showed him what she was doing. She had removed all the tools and boxes from the room and was now in the process of cleaning it up. She had swept the walls and ceiling for cobwebs, and was mopping the floor when he came by.

"Suzy, this looks so much better. If you can keep this up, we will be able to sell the house with no problems. We can use the money to pay your tuition and your rent for an apartment. I am really proud of what you have done here."

"Thanks. I know I have just got started but already I have one room cleared. I hope to have it all done by December," said Suzy.

After her father left, taking the tools he wanted to keep with him, Suzy finished mopping and opened up the shades to let some light into the room. It looked like a completely different place.

After a quick shower, Suzy sat down in front of her TV to catch up on the news. She accomplished a lot of work in a just few days but was wondering if she could keep it up. She didn't do any more work until Saturday, when Martha came over.

When Martha arrived, Suzy proudly showed her the room she had cleared out.

"Suzy, this is wonderful! At this rate it won't be long before we can sell the house and get you moved."

"It was a lot of work, though," said Suzy, "and there were no books in here. It was stuff I really wasn't interested in."

"But, still, you got to work and cleaned it out. It's a great start. What will you work on next?"

"I haven't even thought about that yet. I'm still getting over all the work I did."

"Well, take today and tomorrow off and start again on Monday. How about your bedroom?"

"I don't know. I still use a lot of stuff in there. I think I'll work in the dining room," said Suzy.

"Have you got enough boxes? I can get some more used ones from the firm."

"I think I am going to need as many as I can get for books," answered Suzy.

"I'll bring you some next week," said Martha.

Martha took her out for lunch and told her about the work she was doing. She told Suzy many times that she had the mind of a lawyer and that she, Suzy, would be a good one. Suzy wasn't sure, but now that she was taking her medications regularly, her emotions were certainly under better control and she was much more logical.

After lunch they caught a movie, Martha said it was a reward for all her hard work. They parted company and Suzy spent the rest of the weekend reading and watching television. At Martha's suggestion, she had started getting her books from the library instead of buying them, so they wouldn't clutter up her house anymore. However, she still bought books about bipolar disorder so she could refer to them if she had a question.

Chapter Thirty-Six

On Monday morning, Suzy had her breakfast in the breakfast nook, noticing that fall was coming on, and then walked into the dining room. Every surface was covered. She had a huge job ahead of her. The room was dark and shadowy. No telling what was lurking in the corners. Suzy gave a little shiver. Most of it was books, books stacked on all the chairs, the table and the breakfront. Suzy started to pick them up, dusting them as she looked at them, and putting them in piles. Most of them went into the "keep" pile and after a couple of hours, Suzy found herself getting upset. She asked herself, Why is it fair that I should give up all these things I love so they can sell the house? I have spent my whole life collecting these books and I love them all. I don't want to give away my treasured possessions.

Suzy started to cry and went into the kitchen for a soft drink. She wandered into the living room and sat down in front of the television, not watching or caring what was on. She didn't do any more work that day. She sat around the house, completely idle, unable to put her hand to anything useful. Martha called her that evening, as she usually did, to check on Suzy's progress and to see how she felt. She was surprised that Suzy was cranky and admitted that she hadn't done much work at all that day. "What's wrong, Suzy? What is causing you to have such a bad day?"

"You know I have saved every book I have ever read. I love my books and I don't want to give them up. Father wants to sell the house and I have to give up my favorite things to make him happy."

"Suzy, you aren't thinking clearly. I'm going to stop by for a few minutes on my way home to talk with you. I'll be there soon, and I'll bring you some dinner because I'll bet you haven't thought to eat today."

"No, you don't have to do that. I'll be fine."

"I am going to do it. You need someone right now. I'll be there in a little while."

Suzy didn't want to admit it to herself, but she could use someone to talk with, and food didn't sound like such a bad idea either. She straightened up the kitchen a little and washed her face and combed her hair.

When Martha got there, Suzy was in a somewhat better mood. Martha brought fast food burgers and fries, and Suzy supplied the Diet Cokes. Neither of them often ate fast food, so this was a treat for both of them.

When they finished eating, Martha said, "Show me what tripped you up this morning."

Suzy took her into the dining room and gestured at the piles of books. "I don't know how to give these away."

"You're not thinking clearly. You don't have to keep all these books physically to have access to them. Most of them, and all of the classics, are always available to you from the library. If you give these to the library, you know they will be there. For example, what's this?"

She picked up a book from the pile. "Oh, it's Vonnegut's *Cat's Cradle*. I feel the same way about this book that you do. I don't have a copy of it. If I ever want to reread it, I know there is a copy just waiting for me at the library, and the library will always have this book."

"You are right. I'll only keep my books about bipolar disorder and any books that are special to me, but most of them can go to the library. Thanks. I'll start again in the morning. Now I think I can do it and get the house ready for sale."

The next day Suzy started working again. With only a little backsliding, she was able to clear out the dining room and get it cleaned up in a couple of weeks. She made two trips to the library; she could haul a lot in her pickup. She was grateful that her father had listened to her when she asked him for a truck instead of a car. She made good use of it. With two rooms cleared out Suzy was on a roll, setting a schedule for herself and working steadily to get the house clean. After she tackled the living spaces, she cleared out the attic and the basement. Suzy was surprised to find her stash of pictures of Manny in the attic. She had almost forgotten about them. Of course, she thought of him sometimes and still played his music, but she did not obsess about him as she used to.

Only a few weeks before school started she found an apartment close to school. Just as Martha predicted, her scores on the LSAT were tops and she was admitted with no problem. Martha took the time to go over her freshman texts with her and show her some tricks and some pitfalls before school started. Southern Methodist University wasn't a big, intimidating school. It was a nice size and right in the heart of Dallas. Suzy loved going there and Martha's statement that she had a "lawyer's mind" turned out to be true. Suzy did well in law school and felt her bipolar disorder only during times of stress, such as finals. Then she would sometimes speed up and get a bit irritable, but Martha would help her catch herself before she got out of hand.

She always remembered how paranoid she used to be, and she promised herself she would find a way to do some *pro bono* work for the mentally ill, and especially the homeless mentally ill, when she graduated. She knew she was lucky to have friends, family, and even a great support group to have helped her.

Jackie

Chapter Thirty-Seven

Jackie showed up at school in a blue blazer, grey pants, and black flats. She wanted to make a good first impression by showing off her great figure and her shiny blond hair. She was determined to do well in school to give her a better chance at getting David back.

Richland Junior College is in Richardson, Texas, a suburb of Dallas. It is a small school, known for its good curriculum and excellent teachers. It had a good reputation as a feeder school for the University of Texas. The school's modern buildings were set amid picturesque trees and green spaces, a comfortable place for Jackie to take refuge.

She wasn't sure what to major in, but had the idea of going into journalism. She thought she might be too old to be a newscaster, but even if she didn't make it on TV, there were other options in the field like working behind the scenes or writing for a newspaper or the Internet. During the summer, her counselor told her first to try to test out of some of the basic courses to move herself along a little faster. She hadn't known you could do that, and, with her counselor's help, set up a schedule to take the tests. Jackie was intelligent and well read, and she passed all the tests and received full credit for several basic courses, such as elemental English, history, and Political Science. This gave her an opportunity to take classes that are more advanced and to get ahead.

Several students asked her out, but her requirements were hard to live up to. "No dates on Saturday or Sunday until Sunday night, and no staying out late because I have to study." Most guys weren't willing to go along with this stringent schedule, but the ones who were really interested enough to ask her why, and cared enough to listen to her explanations, heard about her little boy.

"I can see him only on the weekends so I have to keep them free for him. There's nothing more important than that." She was making it difficult, but she had to take care of David first, even though she was lonely and wanted someone to love.

Tom was willing to go along with the requirements to date Jackie. After a while, she was impressed with the creative ways he came up with to spend more time with her. He started having lunch with her daily, even though neither of them had much time for lunch. He asked her, "Where do you study at night? If you go to the library, I could meet you there and we can have our coffee breaks together, even if we can't really study together since we are in different fields." During these short, stolen moments, they found themselves talking and laughing together. They discussed movies, politics, and the price of gas. Jackie found that she was depending on him for company more than she ever realized she would. She was falling in love with him because he was thoughtful and caring.

On a Sunday night, they went to dinner. Afterwards, the weather was just perfect and he drove to a park. They sat on the children's swings and Jackie decided it was time she told him that she had bipolar disorder. Under the stars, with a cool breeze playing through her hair, he listened to her explanation. "It is a mental disorder that is really called a 'mood disorder.' It controls your moods and makes you either sad or happy. I have no control over these moods and it can make me hard to get along with and can make me do things that aren't smart. One of the things I do to combat it is to take medications, which makes me stable and stops the moods from cycling."

Tom said, "So is that why you don't have custody of David?"

"Yes, I gave my parents temporary custody while I was getting on medication and getting straightened out, and they went to court and obtained permanent custody. Even when I got better, they wouldn't return him to me."

"After being around you for these past several months, I can tell you are perfectly sane. At least, as sane as anyone else. I can't believe your parents have done this to you."

"One of the reasons I am going to school is to try to get him back. I have to get good grades and prove that I am capable and responsible so the judge will consider me a good parent. Some of the things I did while I was sick didn't work out so well."

"Jackie, I have all the faith in the world that you can do anything you want to. I don't intend to go anywhere; I'll be with you and I'll help you in any way I can. I don't care if you are crazy; I love you just the same."

"Tom, are you sure you don't want to think about this?"

"No, I am sure. I've seen what you can do and how well you do with David. I'm in for the long haul."

Jackie wanted to spend more time with Tom after this, but she stuck to her schedule, cramming in as much class and study time during the week, working Tom into her days, and then spending as much time as she could on the weekends with David. Jackie thought Tom would get tired of this and go away, but he didn't.

One thing Jackie knew, but wouldn't admit to herself, was that her life was actually easier this way than if she went to school fulltime and was a fulltime mom. Maybe that is why she never pushed for David's return. She complained about her parents having David, but it saved her the cost of a babysitter, of his clothes and food, and the time and attention she would have to give him as she went to school. She also knew that they gave him anything and everything he wanted, and that he might resent her if she pushed until she did get him back, because she could only afford the basics, no expensive video games or name-brand clothing to show off at his private school. She couldn't even afford the private school. She felt defeated whenever she thought of that.

Jackie remained friends with Suzy, even though she lost contact with the other members of the group. She encouraged Suzy and was happy to hear, when she went to law school, how well she was doing. For a while, they met once a month for lunch, but after a while both of their schedules made it impossible and they had to keep up by phone and e-mail. They wondered what had happened to Missy, Marie, Abby, and Carleton, but the only time they got in touch was when the crazy guy shot up the Virginia Tech campus and they all independently checked with Abby with the same message "Are you all right?"

When Jackie finished her two-year course at Richland, she had some basic courses in Journalism and had to make the decision as to which four-year school she would continue her studies in. Her dream had been to go to the University of Texas at Austin, probably the best school open to her, but she knew she would see even less of David if she moved there.

Tom said, "Listen, I will pay for an attorney now to get back custody. You have proven yourself, girl, you've made good grades and demonstrated you could show up on time and finish your classes and take responsibility. I don't think there is a judge in Dallas who would deny you custody of your own son now."

"Tom, I just don't know. I don't want you to spend your money on a lost cause. I'm just not sure at all that I could get David back. He has lived with my parents so long now that I am not at all sure that I could ever get him back."

"Now wait a minute. I am planning to marry you when you get ready. I want you to have your son back and I want us to live as a family. I'm not spending money on you; I'm making an investment in our future."

"I'm just not sure that David is ready for this. He's lived with my parents for years—since he was three. It might be too upsetting to change all his routines now. We need to give him more time." Jackie looked up at Tom beseechingly.

"I don't believe what I am hearing. You don't want David back at all."

"No, Tom, that's not true."

"Then why didn't you jump at my offer to help you get him back? You just want everyone to feel sorry for you because you don't have your child while you are footloose and fancy-free. No babysitters to pay for, no food, no rent for a bigger place, no toys, no expenses at all for you to pay for your boy. You've got it good. I just can't believe it. I really don't want anything more to do with you."

"Tom, no, it's not true. I just want what's best for David. Please don't go." She followed him to the door, but he left without a backward glance. Jackie sank onto the couch and cried. How could he believe such things about her? She was only thinking of David, not herself. This had been her first serious relationship since she was stabilized by medication, and she thought that she deserved the happiness of love. She couldn't believe he walked out on her. Maybe if she waited, he would have second thoughts and come back to her.

Chapter Thirty-Eight

Jackie waited, but Tom did not call her. She couldn't believe that he jumped to such conclusions. It made her so mad she didn't try to call him. Two weeks later, she got a big box from UPS containing everything she left at Tom's apartment. That made her cry again, but Jackie couldn't wallow in her grief. She had too much to do. David was upset that he wouldn't see Tom again, and Jackie comforted him as well as she could. It was like losing his father again. Poor little kid. She had made the right decision to leave him with her parents. He needed the stability there. Tom didn't have the right to walk out on them like that.

The next Monday she spoke to her counselor, "I have definitely decided to continue in Journalism but I am not sure of which school to attend," she said, and gazed wistfully at the brochure from the University of Texas in Austin in her hand, but then thought how much she would miss David if she were that far from him. She knew she would be so busy it would be difficult to get away to see him. Sighing, she set the brochures aside and picked up the information about the University of Texas, Dallas.

Her counselor remarked, "It is a new school and doesn't have the reputation that the Austin campus does, but it has, after all, offered you financial aid. You should also consider the large media market here in Dallas. This is a good source for mentors, internships, and jobs when you graduate. And, of course, you can probably sneak in a visit to David every weekend."

It was a no-brainer. She would go to school in Dallas. Therefore, Jackie enrolled in UT Dallas and started her specialty courses there. She surprised herself by finding that she loved journalism and especially television journalism, but, oddly enough, she didn't like the on-camera work so much. She enjoyed producing. Producing was fast-paced, and she met a lot of different people doing it. She didn't have to spend as much time looking good as she did doing good work. Jackie fell in love with the production end of news, and as part of her classes began doing projects at some of the local media outlets in the city.

She worked with the radio stations, learning timing and clarity and enjoyed meeting the radio personalities she had been listening to all this time. It was fascinating how the behind the scenes operations made everything work so well on the air.

She noticed and mentioned to one early-morning team, "I saw how you signaled each other when you finished talking, so you wouldn't step on each other's words. That explains how radio people can talk with each other so clearly. I never really thought about that before. It was fun watching you throw the ball of dialogue back and forth."

She was happy with her choice of a major, and her teachers considered her a natural. Her media teacher called her in and said, "WFAA, the top TV news station in town, asked for a student for a story they were working on, and I think you would enjoy the assignment and do a good job."

One of the people Jackie got to meet on this assignment was Fred Tisdell, the most well-known reporter in town. He pulled the six o'clock shift on the most popular evening news show. Practically the whole city watched him. He was intelligent, educated, and well-spoken, and surprisingly likable. He wasn't impressed with himself. There was a glimmer between him and Jackie when they met. Neither of them acknowledged it to themselves or to each other.

After the assignment was over, Jackie and Fred started e-mailing each other, about school and the news stories he was doing. Later, they segued into more personal e-mail, and one afternoon he suggested that they meet for a drink at a local club. Jackie was happy; she was nervous as a teenager on a first date. She tried on several outfits, blew off her homework, and drove to the club scared of having a wreck because she could hardly hold onto the wheel. When she got to the club, it was dim inside, but she could pick out Fred immediately. He had the best table in the place and people were dropping by his table to say "hi' all the time. Jackie just watched for a few minutes. He was also the only African-American in the club.

Jackie wasn't sure she wanted to do this. She really liked the guy, but what would her parents think? She knew they would vociferously object to her having any kind of relationship with a black man. She stood there, dithering, for a few minutes, and then thought to herself, it is my life.

She walked over to his table and sat down. He said, "Hello, I'm glad you came."

"I have been looking forward to seeing you again," said Jackie. "You need to catch me up on what you have been doing at work."

"I'll do that, but you need to catch me up on what you've been doing in school."

They laughed, and Jackie said, "I've been working hard, and next semester I will need an internship. I don't suppose you can help with that?"

"I'll do my best to get you one with the station. It will be fun to work together again."

The waiter came to their table.

"Just a minute, what do you want to drink?"

"I want some white wine."

"I'll have the same."

Their conversation took a left turn as they started talking about the war in Iraq and politics. His MA was in Political Science and Jackie followed politics avidly. They soon found that they agreed on almost everything political; that made both of them comfortable. After a seemingly short, but actually long evening of getting to know each other, Fred asked if she would like to take in a dinner and movie next weekend.

"Fred, I can't. My little boy will be at my place for the weekend. I can't date until Sunday night..."

"So you have a little boy and he doesn't live with you?"

"No, he lives with his grandparents and it is a long story. I'll tell you about it sometime."

"You aren't married?"

"No, I am divorced."

"Well, can I take you out on Sunday night?"

"Sure, I just can't stay out too late because I have school."

"And I have a job. It'll work out."

Fred and Jackie became more and more comfortable with each other as they spent more time together. Eventually, Jackie had Fred over on a weekend and let David meet him. David took to him right away, but Jackie told him, "Fred, the shit will hit the fan as soon as David gets home."

When she told him how upset her parents were going to be, he asked, "Won't this make it even more difficult for you to get custody of David?"

"Yes, it will. My parents will fight me tooth and nail, but David has been with them since he was three. They are happy with the situation and David is used to getting all he wants whenever he wants it. Now that they know we are having a relationship, it will be more difficult for me to gain custody. I think it is really for the best. I made that decision before I ever went out with you."

"Really? That is hard to believe. Are you sure, you don't want to pursue this? We can afford it, you know."

"No, I don't want to put David or me through it. We'll all be happier if things remain the same."

Early the next morning, Jackie's phone rang. She saw the call was from her mother and winced.

"Jackie, how could you do this?" her mother asked. "Don't you ever think of anyone but yourself? What will people think of you? What will people think of David? I can't believe you would stoop so low. Do you go out in public with this man? I am ashamed of you."

"Mother, he is a well-educated, well-respected, well-known newsman. In fact, he is the most popular reporter in town. He treats me well and wants to get to know David. I think we have a future together."

"I can't believe this. I am going to go to court and have your visitation annulled."

"Try it, Mother. This is the twenty-first century. You will be laughed out of court."

"Well, don't ask us for any more favors. We are keeping David and I want you to know that I object to that man being around him. We'll have nothing more to do with you."

"If that's the way you want it. But I hope you change your mind in the future and get to know him. You and he would like each other, and Dad would really get along with him."

Click.

~*~

One evening after they edited some tape on a story they had done together, in the dark editing room, Jackie quietly explained her bipolar disorder to Fred. Afterwards, being the understanding, intelligent person he was, he did Internet research until he comprehended all the aspects of it and accepted it.

When Jackie picked up David for his next scheduled visit, he seemed quiet at first. They had dinner with Fred, who then went to the station to get ready for the newscast. Jackie took the day off; it was Friday so she had the whole weekend to spend with David. As soon as Fred left, David started to pepper her with questions, and she could tell where they came from.

"Was it true that Fred won't be able to keep his job long?"

"How did Fred manage living in such a nice house when he probably doesn't make much money?"

"Mom, does he hit you?"

"We never watch him on the news, but Grandma says he doesn't speak English correctly. I know he does, but she won't listen to me."

Jackie answered, "David, I know where you are getting these ideas. Your Grandma is prejudiced against black people and has certain set ideas that are not necessarily correct. You've been around Fred on the weekend and gone places with us; you know what is true. Fred is a good reporter who makes a good salary, and no, you know he doesn't hit me. Now just calm down and don't let your grandma upset you."

"Mom, is there some reason why I can't live with you and Fred?"

"It's just that Grandma and Grandpa have custody of you. Would you like me to try to get custody so you can live with us? You are old enough to choose who you want to live with now."

"Yes, yes I would."

Now that she knew David was on board with the idea, Jackie went to court. With good employment and a happy home life and staying on medication for her bipolar disorder, she was able to regain custody of David with little effort. Fred paid for a lawyer, a Mr. Phipps, who told her it would work out. David happily moved in with them. It took some adjustment on all sides, but eventually they even managed to set up visitation with Jackie's parents who missed David so much they forced themselves to be civil to Fred.

Now Jackie had David back, and she had Fred's love. She was stable with her bipolar disorder. Things had worked out for her better than she ever thought they would, back when she wrecked her car and was committed to the hospital.

Missy

Chapter Thirty-Nine

Missy couldn't believe the nerve of those two continuously telling her to keep taking the pills, keep doing something that had no upside. She put on a happy face for Tyrone when she got to the car in the parking lot of the Denny's, but she was pissed off inside. They went to her place, had sex as they normally did, and then she asked him to leave her alone. "I need to think for a while, Tyrone."

She was sick of it all. Of taking those pills whose only effect was to mess up her mind, steal her words, and make her skin crawl. They weren't helping. Neither were all the people who thought they were so superior telling her to "keep trying, keep trying." She was tired of trying and not getting anywhere, and she saw no reason to continue. She was also feeling restless, like there wasn't any excitement in her life, and she needed something exciting to happen. She knew she needed a change.

Missy went into the bathroom and picked up all her pills. It took both hands to hold them all. She couldn't believe she had fallen for the doctors, nurses, and support group members who tried to convince her that these would actually make her feel better. She looked in the mirror and saw Missy looking back at her. Missy had bright eyes, and when she smiled, a happy face. She didn't need all those useless pills. She lined the pill bottles up on the area around the sink and one by one, took off the lids (that was another thing—who came up with those rotten safety lids!) and poured the contents down the toilet. Flushing it was the last step.

Now she was free of all that advice and all that medication that didn't make her feel any better. She could

go back to being her true self. Just to make certain, she
blocked the phone numbers of all the members of the group
on her phone and unfriended them from her Facebook page.
Now, she wouldn't have to listen to them anymore. They
didn't know what went on inside her head, even though
they said they did.

She called Tyrone and asked him to pick her up that
night. She had been careful until then to live her life
carefully, as she was advised, staying away from liquor,
which the group and her doctor told her was bad for her and
would interfere with her meds. When he got to her place,
she asked him to take her to a club. They went, and Missy
drank vodka all evening. She felt free, free of all the
constraints that had been put on her by her mother, her
doctors, and the group.

She didn't think about going back to work—she had
steady income from disability and that would keep her in
her apartment, and in liquor. She could feel herself
loosening up. However, Tyrone wasn't too happy with the
way things were going. He did not want to spend his time
drinking and clubbing. When he met Missy, she was
attempting to get well and living a sedate life. He didn't
like the new Missy who drank and wanted to stay up half
the night.

After a couple of nights of going to the club, he asked,
"Missy, can't we stay home tonight? I'd rather just watch
television. There are some good shows on. And you know I
have to go to work in the morning."

"No, of course not. I want to go out and have fun.
What are you, an old stick in the mud? If you won't take
me out, I'll just find someone who will."

"Missy, don't do that. I thought we had something
special."

"Not anymore. Now, just leave. I have some
arrangements to make."

"Missy…."

"No, go. I want you out of here. Now."

Tyrone reluctantly left her apartment, and Missy called the club they went to the night before. She already had an eye on a guy there and got him on the phone. She explained who she was, described herself to him, and he was happy to drive over and pick her up. Missy dove into the club scene, back to drinking a bottle of vodka a night and sleeping all day.

She could not believe it when, a week later, the cops knocked on her door in the middle of the day to tell her that those stupid people, Carleton and Marie, were worried about her. Just because she didn't show up for their little meeting didn't mean that there was anything wrong with her, for God's sake. She was polite to the policeman, but she made it quite clear that she wanted nothing more to do with those two.

"I am doing just fine. Tell those people I don't want to see or hear from them again." Maybe they'd get the message and leave her alone.

The new man she hooked up with, Jermaine, didn't mind spending his time at clubs at all. He worked at a car dealership, readying cars for delivery. He delighted in Missy's quest for fun and matched her drink for drink, until she went over the top. She even complained that she was too high to enjoy herself, and Jermaine told her he could help by giving her a pill. "Well, I don't know if I want any pills, Jermaine. I've pretty much had my fill of them."

"No, these will chill you out, make you feel good. Just one or two a day and you are good."

"Okay, let me try one."

Missy took one, and soon felt a smoothing out, a disconnection from the travails of daily life. She felt a calmness, a slowing down of her jumpy brain. She felt like she was floating away from all her troubles. She even went to sleep for a while. Missy hadn't been able to sleep for several days, so it was a real relief. She felt so much better when she woke up.

"Jermaine, that was great. Can you get more of those?"

"Sure, I might have to have you pony up for some of them, but I have a supplier."

"Jermaine, I won't get addicted to these, will I?"

"Nah, not if you just take one or two a day."

"Okay, they really helped me. I have such a hard time sleeping. Now I feel like making love. Those pills are great."

"And if you like them so much, I'll make sure you have plenty of them."

Missy and Jermaine happily continued their relationship, but Missy wanted more and more of the pills. When she asked Jermaine what they were, he said, "OxyContin." That made Missy stop for a minute. She heard about people becoming addicted to that drug and ruining their lives. Nevertheless, she thought, no way was that going to happen to her.

As the weeks passed, Missy started needing more and more of the pills to get that blissed-out feeling she needed. When she got up to ten pills a day, Jermaine tried to put the brakes on.

"Missy, that many pills aren't good for you. You aren't taking them anymore to feel good; you are taking them because you need them. You'll never be able to get enough unless you stop now. It'll just get worse and worse. I'm cutting you back to two a day right now. It's for your own good."

Missy tossed her head and said, "So you think you are the only guy who can get pills? I don't need you. I'll get my own."

"Missy, don't do this. You will be sorry you started this. Let me help you before it is too late."

"Jermaine, the reason I met you is that I got tired of people preaching at me. I can take care of myself. Just leave. I'm good. You take things too seriously."

"Missy, I'm only trying to help you. You need to get off those pills before bad things happen to you."

"You know what? Everyone who has been preaching to me the past few weeks has been trying to help me. Well, I don't need any help, for your information. I am just fine, and I'll be even better when you get out."

"I'll leave, but call me when you need help—and you will need help. I wish you would listen to me now."

"Good-bye, Jermaine."

Jermaine left, sorry that he had ever given her pills. He truly cared about her and hated to see her go down this road. He knew she would wind up miserable and alone, but hoped she would remember to call him then.

Chapter Forty

Missy knew right where to start to find another man, another supply. There was a guy at the club who flirted aggressively, sending her a clear message. She called the club that night and asked, "Could I speak to Jackson?"

Missy said 'hello' to Jackson and he knew who she was. He countered with a big 'hello' and said, "What can I do for you?"

Missy replied, "I am sitting at home all alone and bored. I wondered if you might want to come over and bring me to the club."

Jackson said, "I sure would. Give me your address."

Missy gave him directions to her apartment and he hurried right over and picked her up. Missy greeted him, then cut to the chase and asked him, "Do you know how to get OxyContin?"

"Sure, baby, I can get you any amount, any time."

"Like now?"

"Let's go."

Jackson drove her to an unfamiliar neighborhood called Oak Cliff in Dallas. He went into a house while she sat in the truck, and came out in a few minutes with a stash of pills. They both took some and went on to the club, where Missy had her usual vodka. The vodka and the pills took the edge off her manic high and she felt less irritable and abrasive.

Jackson came over afterwards and there was no question they would have sex. Then he just sort of hung around. After he had been with her for a couple of weeks, one night he didn't come home. Missy met him at the door the next morning with a voice like sandpaper. "Where were you last night?"

"What difference does it make? I left you well-supplied, just like you always have food in the house for me. What I do with my nights is my business."

"I can't believe you would just stay out all night without even calling me. I didn't know if you were hurt or what."

"You want me to leave?"

"No, no, I don't."

"Good, because I brought you some pills."

It didn't matter to Missy. She only needed him because he was her source of supply.

They took some pills and went to bed. After they had been asleep for a couple of hours, Missy heard knocking at the door. She ignored it. Then came a loud banging. Cursing under her breath, Missy went to the door and answered it. To her surprise, it was her mother. Missy had been putting off her mother for several weeks because she didn't want her to see how she looked. She didn't think she looked her best.

Her mother said, "Missy what is going on with you? You haven't called me for a ride to the doctor's or anywhere else for weeks. What have you been doing?"

"Well, Mom, you know, the doctors really weren't doing me all that much good, so I quit going."

"So you have stopped your therapy?"

"Yes."

"From the looks of you, you are taking drugs. And who is this?"

"Oh, I'm sorry, this is Jackson. He is my boyfriend."

"Why are you all in bed in the middle of the afternoon? Don't answer that. I know what is going on. Missy, don't come to me for help. I told you about Blanche and you are headed the same way she went. I won't help you get there. I can't tell you how sad it makes me to hear you say you are giving up."

"Mom, I'm not giving up. Aunt Blanche and I have nothing in common. I'm doing just fine. And I won't come to you for help because I don't need any help."

"I hope you come to your senses and that I see you again."

"Bye, Mom."

Her mother slowly backed out of the door, looking at Missy as if she could never get her fill of seeing her; as if it was the last time she would ever see her.

"Jackson, everyone I know except you is all concerned about my business. That's why you and I get along. You just want to have a good time, like me."

Life went along at the apex for six months. Slowly, though, Missy began to lose steam. Drinking and drugging began to lose their appeal. She wasn't happy all the time. It seemed to her that the world had somehow become a dark, dreary place. She was a real drag on Jackson, who was still up for fun and games twenty-four seven.

Missy spent more time in bed, but took more pills to sleep. She wouldn't go out clubbing; she just didn't enjoy it anymore. She stopped drinking. It didn't make her feel better anymore. She looked at herself in the mirror, a gaunt wraith, marred with acne, shaggy hair, and raccoon eyes peered back at her. Now she knew what her mother was looking at when she visited. Though it didn't really matter what she looked like, she was more concerned with how she felt. It wasn't good.

She cashed her check that month and carefully set back the rent money—she learned from the last time she went through one of these phases. However, Jackson was bored with her now; she was no fun. He decided to take his truck and find someone who wanted to be with him. He thought it would be easier if he had a little cash, so he took Missy's rent money when he left.

It took Missy a couple of days to realize he was gone. She was in a depression, augmented by the pills. Finally, she woke up in a morning with no more pills and no money. She checked her rent-money stash, because she somehow had to get pills, and discovered it was gone. She knew where it went.

Slowly it came to Missy that she had hit a dead end. She had no transportation, no food, no drugs, and no money. Helpless and scared, she no longer felt that she could conquer the world. Missy waited until evening. It was dark when she set out, about 6:00 p.m. It wasn't too cold; the high that day was forecast in the seventies. Without bus money, she had to walk to her mother's house.

It was so dry there was dust on the bushes beside the sidewalk and little poofs of dust came up where she stepped where there wasn't a sidewalk. Missy was shaking and she had to stop to vomit several times. The darkness hid her from the neighbors and from herself. When she got to the familiar door, she knocked, and her mother answered. "Mom, I know you said not to come here, but Jackson stole all my money and I have nothing. I need money for food and rent and to take the bus."

"Missy, what did I tell you? You won't get any help from me. Until you are off drugs and ready to go back to the doctor and take your medication, I will not help you. I know you think I am cruel, but I never told you who found Blanche's body. I couldn't go through that again. It makes me sad, but I simply can't help you."

She shut the door. Out of Missy's sight, she slowly slid down the wall until she was sitting on the floor. She brought her apron to her eyes and wept inconsolably.

Missy went to the neighbor's and asked for a drink. The lady had known her all her life, but she had never seen her so rough looking. Seeing Missy like that kind of scared her, but she gave her an ice-cold glass of water and told her she was happy to see her. Missy said, "Thank you," and started down the street back to her apartment.

She dialed her phone as she walked and when someone answered, she said, "Jermaine?"

Marie

Chapter Forty-One

Even though she was directionally disabled, Marie caught on as to how the streets were laid out in Dallas. After a few months, she was tooling around like a native. She lived in the north part of town, and soon learned that the north-south artery was the Tollway. That made it easier to find places.

Marie always had that one close girlfriend who she could share things with and she missed that relationship in Dallas. She had no concrete plans for finding such a friend. Friends like that usually sneaked up on you when you weren't looking for them. On a hot afternoon while running errands she stopped at the local convenience store for an icy drink and saw a stack of Avon booklets lying on the counter.

She asked the clerk, "Are you giving those out?"

The clerk replied, "They are there for anyone who wants one. Take one if you want."

She missed having access to Avon goodies and so took a booklet. That evening, back in the air conditioning, she paged through the book and found some things she wanted to order. She filled out the order blank and left the envelope for the postman. Then she forgot about it.

A couple of weeks later, the Avon lady called. "Your order has come in. When would it be convenient for me to bring it by?" It took Marie a moment to remember what she was talking about.

"Oh, I am home most of the time or I can come by your place and pick it up. Whatever is most convenient for you."

"No, I'll drop it off at your apartment. I know where you live."

About an hour later, an attractive, tall blonde woman brought her order over. They sat down to talk. Marie found her friendly and they were getting along well. She found out that her name was Penny Ride, and they had a lot in common, including their ages.

As they were talking, Marie was playing a CD and Penny asked about it. Marie said,

"Guess what? I am friends with the Four Preps, who I knew when I was a teenager. Of course, now they are an oldies group. The lead singer told me to check out his daughters' music and I just got their CD. I like it so much that I wanted you to hear one of the songs."

The song was *Moonblind*, by his daughter, Tracey, written for a friend of hers who had AIDS. As the song played, Marie was startled to see Penny pull out a handkerchief and wipe her eyes.

"What's wrong, Penny?"

"That song, it's so moving."

Suddenly they were talking to each other about anything and everything.

After a couple of hours of nonstop talking, they discovered they only lived a block or so from one another. Penny said, "We are so close, I want you to come over for dinner tomorrow night. I want to introduce you to my son. Now, come over about 5:30, because we eat early."

"Good," said Marie, I'll be there." All the next day she looked forward to a quiet evening at her new friend's home.

The next evening she walked down the street to Penny's house. She was surprised to find that Penny lived not only with her son, Aaron, but also with her ex-husband, Jimmy. Jimmy had fallen on hard times and Penny had taken him in when he needed a place to stay.

Penny asked, "Is Chinese okay?"

Marie answered, "Sure."

Penny said, "What do you like?"

Marie said, "Orange chicken is my favorite."

"Good, that's my favorite, too. The guys can have whatever they want. We'll split an order."

Aaron was quiet, but Jimmy was friendly and talkative. Marie was impressed that everyone got along so well, especially when Penny's boyfriend came over later in the evening. She thought that Penny and her family were one of the more civilized families she had ever met.

After this, Marie visited during the day, when Jimmy was at work and Aaron was at school so she could have long conversations with Penny. When she finally wanted to tell Penny she had bipolar disorder, she hesitated, afraid of losing her new best friend, who she sorely needed. They were sitting on the patio, sipping cold drinks in the morning. Slowly twisting a piece of hair through her fingers, she finally spoke.

"Penny, I need to tell you something. I have bipolar disorder and that's why I don't work and have applied for disability."

"So? I take Prozac for depression and I'm on disability for my back, which got hurt in a car wreck. I'm sorry I can't work anymore, but them's the breaks. How is your application going?"

"Slowly, I have been denied twice and now I'm waiting for a hearing. It's scary because all the money I have is from the sale of my house. I have a lawyer, but he says we just have to wait. I don't know what I'll do if I don't get disability—I can't seem to get a job at my age."

"Well, we'll work on it together. Really, the major thing we have to worry about is our old cars giving out."

"That's the truth," said Marie.

Marie's lawyer, Mr. Brice, contacted her when the hearing date was set. "Now don't dress like you are going to work, and get someone to drive you to the hearing. Don't wear makeup or fix your hair. Try to look somewhat pitiful."

Marie told Penny about that and she volunteered to drive Marie. The morning of the hearing, Marie put on a T-shirt and pants that had really been cute fifteen years ago, but now were faded and washed out. She fixed her hair, but didn't spray it, so it would fall in a couple of hours, and put on minimum make-up.

Marie's stomach was upset the day of the hearing because she so needed the income and she really didn't think she would be able to work; she had lost so many jobs in the past. When they were called into the hearing, the Social Security Judge looked at Marie's records, and then said, "I have already come to a decision in this case."

Marie's lawyer kicked her under table, hard. Marie assumed that meant not to say anything. The Judge went on, "It is obvious that this woman can't hold a job, she has had so many of them and so many periods of unemployment. Therefore, I am awarding disability to her to start this month."

Marie and the Mr. Brice thanked the judge and got out of there. Marie thanked the lawyer for doing all the paperwork. Penny was startled to see them come out of the hearing room so quickly. Marie explained that she didn't even have a hearing, and Penny laughed. Then she and Penny went to a pizza place to celebrate. "Now you at least know you will have shelter and food," said Penny.

"Yes, that is a big worry lifted off me. It's not much, but I won't be homeless, and I will try to get into subsidized housing."

"I didn't want to tell you this, but now that you know you are settled, I will. Jimmy is back on his feet and moving into his own place, and now that Aaron has graduated, he is going with him. I don't have anyone to help with the rent and bills, so I am moving in with my brother, Tom, who lives in Arlington"

"Penny, I will miss you so much! I can't believe you are moving so far away."

"We can still talk on the phone, but it won't be the same as when you could just walk down the street."

After Penny left, Marie missed her a lot, but got busy finding a subsidized apartment and getting moved. It was sad not to be working anymore, but she really felt that she couldn't, not after what had happened at MedPrime, and given her age. Therefore, she resigned herself to writing for herself and doing all the reading she desired.

Chapter Forty-Two

Since Marie had only written for political and medical training companies previously, she knew little about writing a memoir, so she joined a local writing group for help and encouragement. With the help of the group, writing the memoir wasn't hard at all. It was liberating to admit on paper that she suffered from bipolar disorder.

She didn't have to worry about her employer seeing it with disability to live on. It only took six months to get it all down. Writing as fast as she could, sometimes waking up in the middle of the night to jot something down. The title came from a song written by Tracey, *Fire and Ice*. She felt it was particularly appropriate in defining bipolar disorder. She used it with Tracey's permission.

After finishing it, she researched how to get published then spent six months trying to find an agent, receiving piles of rejection letters. Everything was returned to her, always with the notation there was no interest in that type of book. Marie knew better, but didn't know how to connect with the right people. Next, she tried the publishers of other bipolar memoirs, but nothing worked. Finally, a member of her writing group, Neil, suggested, "Why don't you self-publish?"

"What is that?" Marie asked.

"There are companies who will publish your book. You retain all the rights, and they will print and distribute it."

Marie so badly wanted her book out there, available to others with bipolar disorder, she decided to do it that way. She knew she could help others with her story. She paid a company to bring it out and then did some publicity, not much, on her own. To her surprise, her book caught on and strictly by word of mouth started selling. She received many emails from people who were grateful for the book, and she didn't mind that it meant that she was coming completely out of the closet as far as her writing group was concerned. From there she volunteered to write grant proposals for a nonprofit group that sponsored book festivals. Writing kept her busy and from being so lonely. Feeling better, she started to make new friends.

At the behest of the book festival organization, she created a Facebook page. Her first friends were the book festival people, but then she added MedPrime employees and relatives. Soon she had over a hundred friends she was keeping up with, including Abby and Carleton. She enjoyed it more than she ever thought possible and it gave her another way to connect to the world.

She kept up with the singing group she was friends with through their website and email and even went to some of their shows. They were popular when she was a teenager and could still pull in an enormous crowd, though now a much older one. It was great that they remained so popular. She wasn't dating anyone and hadn't for years, but she was happy with her life situation. She was feeling stable and able to take life as it came.

When the phone rang after midnight, she automatically answered it, half-groggy. The person on the line was speaking so fast she could not make out the words. She said, "Whoa, I can't understand you; slow down."

"It's Carleton."

"Carleton? Are you all right? Why are you talking so fast? Slow down."

She made out, "I want to come and see you. I love you," he said with extreme enunciation.

"Carleton, you are manic. You need to go to a doctor. You don't love me, and you can't come see me. We are just friends."

"No, I love you. I want to move in with you."

"Carleton, there is no way. Go straight to the clinic in the morning. You are way manic. You are not thinking straight. Now, goodbye." Marie hung up the phone.

Marie was wide-awake and upset. Carleton was never any more than a friend. A manic person showing up on her doorstep was the last thing she needed. She thought briefly of trying to find him and keeping him safe until the clinic opened in the morning but realized that she didn't have a clue as to where he was, and she really didn't want to get involved. Instead, she blocked his number on her cellphone and unfriended him on her Facebook page. There. Now he wouldn't be able to get in touch with her. He didn't have her address, so he couldn't come over.

Marie would not have her own sanity disturbed by this person who had never seemed to be able to get it together. Marie always said that she wished to help others, but it was too much to ask her to rescue someone who would just be in the same shape in a few months. She wanted to help them with her writing, not getting involved with them as individuals. She couldn't help him without risking the life she had made for herself. Nothing was worth that.

Marie deliberately set out to forget about the call and the whole incident. She never mentioned it to anyone or thought about it again. It was settled. She was fine.

Carleton

Chapter Forty-Three

Carleton did not confide in people. He found that they generally did not take it well, and would-be friends disappeared from his life. In this case, he chanced it. His next-door neighbor, Bill Pogue, had been friendly with him since he moved in a couple of years ago. They had started hanging out, watching movies together and sharing their life stories. Bill was short and stocky, with long, flowing blond hair. He always wore a big turquoise pendant, a silver and turquoise cuff, and a turquoise ring.

Finally, when they were talking in Bill's apartment, Carleton said, "You know, I have this problem with bipolar disorder."

"Really?" said Bill. "What's that like?"

"I have bipolar disorder. It causes me to lose control of my mood and go manic. That means I get really, really happy and do some strange things. I talk fast, and walk fast, play music too fast, and may spend too much money. If you ever see me acting like this, just please stay away from me."

Bill said, "That sounds odd. I'll do that."

Later on, Bill, who had an uncle with bipolar disorder, decided to learn more about it. Whenever people in his family talked about his Uncle Ross, they used hushed tones and wouldn't discuss what was wrong with him. It seemed mysterious to Bill when he was a child, and now he decided to demystify it since he had a neighbor with the same disorder.

He simply searched for "bipolar disorder" on Google and got dozens of results. He read about it all afternoon. He could see why it was difficult to live with and why people had trouble dealing with people who had it, but it didn't scare him. That weekend, he went to the library and got two books about it. He skimmed them and then brought the subject up again with Carleton the next time he saw him.

"Carleton, I read about bipolar disorder and I can see why it messes up your life, but if you need help anytime, don't hesitate to ask me. I learned a lot about it and while I know it is difficult for you, I wouldn't mind helping you at all."

"Thanks, Bill, for the offer, but I hope I would never have to involve you. I wouldn't want to make you mad or upset you in any way. When I am manic I am a different person and I don't want you to see me that way."

"Don't worry about it. Understanding it makes all the difference. Don't ever hesitate to ask me if you need something."

"Okay."

Carleton was embarrassed, but he asked, "Hey, I heard today that *Lincoln* has finally hit the cheap theatre in the neighborhood. Do you want to try to catch the matinêe?"

"Sure, let's go."

Their relationship continued as before, but the subject of bipolar disorder never came up again. Bill was curious and wanted to ask questions, but it was obvious that Carleton didn't want to talk about it. Bill was also a musician, so they both worked odd hours, though Bill got more work than Carleton did, but they sometimes had time to hang out together. They spent a lot of time in Bill's apartment, watching movies and TV and just shooting the bull.

Late on a weekday night, someone rapped loudly on Bill's door. When Bill didn't immediately answer the knock, the rap came again, louder. Bill opened the door, thinking there was some kind of emergency. It was just Carleton wanting to visit. Bill let him in. At first, something seemed off, and then Bill realized that he was talking faster than he usually did. He kept pacing around the apartment, not wanting to sit down. He was barefoot. Bill couldn't put his finger on what was going on.

He asked Carleton, "Hey, what's wrong with you?"

"There's nothing wrong with me." Carleton said. "What makes you think there's something wrong with me?"

"I don't know...you just don't seem yourself to me tonight."

"I'm fine, everything's normal. Am I bothering you?"

"No, not at all. It's just making me a little nervous that you won't sit down."

"I just don't feel like sitting down. I've got too much energy tonight. Don't know why, but I really feel good."

Carleton started to tell Bill stories about things that happened to him in the past, but he could never seem to stay on the subject or get to the point. "I had this girlfriend in L.A. who was really pretty. You should have seen her, long black hair and big brown eyes. One night we went out and while we were out we met her girlfriend, and man, she was a looker and later on I started dating her and she had this big, black dog that I was afraid of at first, but he turned out to be a sweetheart and then I got way happy and lost my job..."

Suddenly it clicked for Bill. Carleton was well into a manic state. From the little he knew, he thought he shouldn't leave Carleton alone to get into trouble. He thought he would stay with him and see if it got any worse. He sat with him and pretended to listen to his ramblings.

"Carleton, will you stay with me tonight? I don't want to be alone."

Carleton said cheerfully, "Sure, I don't have a job tonight. I want to talk to you anyway."

As it got later, Bill found himself less and less able to keep up with Carleton's meandering talk. At some point, he must have dozed off, because he came to just as Carleton was hanging up the phone. "Hey buddy, you don't need to be calling people at this time of night. Who was that, anyway?"

"Oh, just a girl. I thought she might want to go out with me but I guess not."

"Well, just stay off the phone until morning. It's after two."

"Okay."

Getting his second wind, Bill was able to observe Carleton for a while. He seemed to be even more speeded up, and clumsier. "Say, have you taken your medication tonight?" asked Bill

"Don't know. I don't think I need it anyway. I feel really good."

"I can see that. I'm really getting hungry. Why don't we go next door and get some shoes, and then go to Denny's for some breakfast. Does that sound like a good deal?"

"Yeah, it does, though I don't know why I need shoes."

"Well, you know, 'no shoes, no service.'"

"Yep, better get some shoes."

With that, they went to Carleton's apartment and he slipped into a pair of loafers, not bothering with socks. Bill noted that the apartment was a mess. On the way out to the car, Carleton talked loudly about going to Denny's, and Bill said, "Shh, Carleton, people are trying to sleep, and we sure don't want anyone to call the police."

"Well, why would they do that?"

"Because you are making so much noise."

"Oh, sorry."

Bill's mind was not on what Carleton was talking about as he drove, but he tried to sound like he was listening. When they got to the hospital, Carleton said, "Why are we stopping here? This isn't Denny's."

"I have a friend here and I promised I would bring him something. Come on in—you will like him."

"Okay."

When they got to the admitting office, Carleton was still rambling on about his life and didn't seem to notice his surroundings. Bill spoke quietly to the admitting nurse, saying, "My friend Carleton is in a manic state and I think he needs some care."

Carleton was reading notices on the bulletin board aloud, but not really comprehending what was happening. "The summer picnic for staff will be held on Saturday, May 11, 2013 at San Gabriel River Park. The nurse's book club is not meeting during the summer months."

The nurse called someone on the phone and spoke softly, "We need Dr. Brown at Admitting, STAT."

Carleton, suddenly curious about what the nurse was doing, asked Bill, "Aren't we going to see your friend?"

Bill answered, "In a minute, buddy, I've got something to take care of first."

"What would you have to take care of in a hospital? Wait a minute, I think you are trying to shanghai me—oh no, you don't!"

Carleton turned and started for the door. Bill intercepted him, just as Dr. Brown arrived.

The doctor did a quick examination, talking quietly and calmly he asked Carleton, "How are you feeling tonight? Have you been doing anything special?"

Carleton answered him loudly and rapidly, "I feel really good, I have just been talking to my friend, Bill, tonight." His speech was pressured or rapid and forced and his mania was obvious.

Dr. Brown said, "I think you need to stay here for a while and take some medication. It is not safe for you to leave."

Carleton, again loudly and rapidly, stated, "There is nothing wrong with me." He turned to Bill, saying, "I can't believe you lied to me, man."

Bill said, "Believe me, I am only trying to help you. Call me when you need a ride home."

"I will never speak to you again," Carleton said as he turned and followed the doctor down the hall.

Chapter Forty-Four

When Carleton got home from the hospital, he was depressed. He took a Yellow Cab home, not wanting to call Bill for help. Shortly after he returned home, Bill knocked on his door. Carleton watched him through the peephole, but didn't answer. He didn't want to talk to him, embarrassed that Bill had seen him manic and out of control. He was still angry that Bill tricked him into going to the hospital, even though it had stopped his mania before it got any worse.

Carleton just sat and thought about his life. He would never get any better; he was doomed always to succumb to periodic bouts of mania. He would always screw up his life, lose jobs, and ruin relationships by going high as a kite every year or so. He remembered the easy camaraderie of the group, where everyone was equal and people laughed at his jokes. They listened to him and took his problem seriously. He also remembered their promises—that they would always be his friends. Flying buttresses, indeed, he snorted. They had offered him no support. Now they wouldn't answer his e-mails, and Marie wouldn't even talk to him on the phone when she realized he was manic. He didn't recall what he said to her, but he knew she had ended the call early and he couldn't get a hold of her after that. It was the story of his life. Nothing was ever going to get better, no matter what he tried or how hard he worked at it.

He had been given this great talent to make music but his disorder even fouled that up. You would think that would be something he could count on. But no, occasionally his talent was sabotaged and he would lose his ability to make music, losing his job as a consequence. He lived to make music and even that was taken away from him. He had nothing.

Was there any use in continuing? He knew his future, and he didn't want to live in it. He didn't really believe in life after death, so it just meant leaving this life, which was the only one he would ever have. He just didn't know why he was singled out for this awful disorder that kept him alone, why, he couldn't even have a kitten. Since his mother's death, nothing or no one loved him and never would. He saw no use in staying alive. He would just be unhappy until the day he died, and God knew what he would have to go through before that happened. It just didn't seem worth it to keep trying.

He straightened up the apartment, still thinking. He picked up, washed the dishes, made the bed, and generally got things in order. He was kind of messy when he was manic. He didn't see the point in washing clothes, though. After his housekeeping chores, he checked on his stash. He had several kinds of medications he had tried over the years, plus a good amount of lithium. He also had some pain pills he had been prescribed when he had that migraine. He hadn't bothered to take all of them but had saved them in case he needed them for another migraine or some other pain-related problem. He had some sleeping pills, and the nurse had told him not to mix them with another prescription she had given him for akthisia, a form of anxiety that required him to keep moving. That sounded promising.

Carleton gathered all the pills into one place, then sat and looked at them. He wondered if there was anything else he needed to do. He decided to delete some personal correspondence from his computer, which took only minutes. Then he decided to write a suicide note; people should know why he'd done it. He actually got pretty carried away with it. It turned into an indictment of people who treated mentally ill people badly and raged against the stigma of mental illness that many people held. He read it over and wondered if he should tone it down as it had turned into a rant. But, hey, it was how he really felt and it couldn't embarrass him after he was dead, so he left it.

Again, he thought of his reason for suicide, and again he saw no reason to go on living. His life was a burden to him and he couldn't bear it any longer. With no belief in a life after death, he assumed that life after his death would be a whole lot like his life before birth. He didn't remember being sad or hurt or embarrassed or manic during that time. Therefore, he would just be trading all the pain of his present life for nothingness. Right then, it seemed like a good trade.

He happened to have some vodka in the refrigerator that Bill had given him after a party he went to. Carleton hadn't felt like drinking it, but it would be a great chaser for the pills.

It was evening when he started taking the pills, in no order, drinking the vodka as he swallowed them. He took them in handfuls, putting as many as fifteen pills in his mouth and then washing them down with a swig of vodka. Soon he got groggy, but he kept on taking pills and drinking. He didn't know when he lost consciousness.

~~*~~

When he opened his eyes, all he knew was that the sun was shining directly in them and it hurt. He didn't know anything else. He was confused and didn't know why he was lying on the couch. There was vomit on the floor and he really wondered why he had made such a mess. He didn't remember it.

Then it came back to him. His first feeling was of relief that he didn't die. He wasn't certain what that would have been like, but at least he knew what life was like. He was scared by what he had almost done. Still groggy, he knew what he had done and that he had not succeeded. He had returned to the world he was familiar with and he knew how it worked, even though it left him unhappy much of the time. For the first time in a long time, life seemed precious to him. Thirsty, after a while he got a drink of water. He sat back down immediately.

For two hours he sat, letting his head clear and gathering his strength, not believing what he had done. His life was the pits, but it was all he had. Maybe he would try getting a kitten again after all.

He decided he would find a hospital that would work with him to try to break his manic cycle. Maybe he didn't have to live like this for the rest of his life. Maybe there was a way to solve his basic problem. The least he could do was to try. He should have done that before trying to kill himself. After he cleaned up the mess, he was going to start an inquiry on Google to see if he could find a place that was researching mania to try to get some help. He would start with NIH. It wasn't right just to give up.

When he was able to move around again, he tore the suicide note into tiny pieces, threw it into the trash, and got a Diet Coke, which helped settle his messed-up stomach. He looked at the clock and saw it was ten a.m. The whole day stretched out before him; "Well," he said to himself, "I guess I'll go next door and talk to Bill."

www.ingramcontent.com/pod-product-compliance
Lightning Source LLC
Chambersburg PA
CBHW051449170526
45166CB00001B/174